THE INTERNATIONAL PHARMACOPOEIA

THIRD EDITION

VOLUME 1

GENERAL METHODS OF ANALYSIS

THE INTERNATIONAL PHARMACOPOEIA

THIRD EDITION

PHARMACOPOEA INTERNATIONALIS

EDITIO TERTIA

Volume 1

General Methods of Analysis

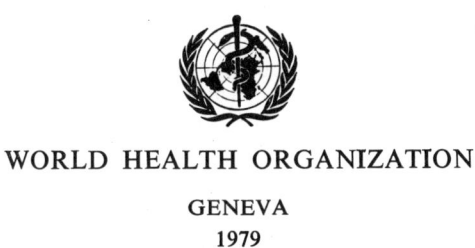

WORLD HEALTH ORGANIZATION

GENEVA

1979

ISBN 92 4 154150 4

PRINTED IN FRANCE

78/3944 — 9000 — BERGER-LEVRAULT

CONTENTS

BIOLOGICAL METHODS

METHODS OF PHARMACOGNOSY

MISCELLANEOUS

PREFACE

The *International Pharmacopoeia* is published by the World Health Organization by virtue of resolution WHA3.10[1] of the Third World Health Assembly. The first edition was published in two volumes, the first in 1951 and the second in 1955, followed by a Supplement in 1959; all of these were issued in English, French and Spanish. German and Japanese translations have also been published. The second edition was published in 1967, followed by a Supplement in 1971. These were issued in English, French, Russian and Spanish.

The WHO Expert Committee on Specifications for Pharmaceutical Preparations, in its 25th and 26th reports, has reviewed the organization of work on the revision of the *International Pharmacopoeia* and on the production and review of quality specifications published by the World Health Organization. It recommended suitable procedures and established priorities with a view to the implementation of World Health Assembly resolutions WHA20.34,[2] which requested the Director-General "to continue work on analytical control specifications", and WHA28.66,[3] which requested the Director-General "to continue to develop activities related to the establishment and revision of international standards, requirements and guidelines for prophylactic and therapeutic substances".

Following these recommendations, work has been proceeding on the preparation of the third edition of the *International Pharmacopoeia*, which will be published in several volumes. Volume 1 contains the description of general methods of analysis; it will be followed by volumes containing the monographs, i.e., quality specifications for individual drugs, primarily for those most widely used in general health care.

The selection of the methods and procedures included in volume 1 of the third edition was based on their utility for the purpose of assuring the quality of pharmaceuticals. Numerous alterations have been made in the methods retained from previous editions to bring them into line with progress in the development of new analytical tools. Full account was, however, taken of various technical and economic constraints, and in the choice of recommended procedures optimum solutions were sought that will, it is hoped, permit their use by drug quality control laboratories located in developing countries as well.

---

[1] *WHO Handbook of Resolutions and Decisions*, vol. I, 1973, p. 127.
[2] *WHO Handbook of Resolutions and Decisions*, vol. I, 1973, p. 132.
[3] *WHO Handbook of Resolutions and Decisions*, vol. II, third edition, 1979, p. 52.

The revision of the general methods of analysis included in Volume 1 of the third edition was carried out with the help of the members of the WHO Expert Advisory Panel on the International Pharmacopoeia and Pharmaceutical Preparations and other specialists. The process of revision was carried out in a series of meetings held during the period 1974-1977 and by correspondence. In July 1978 the draft text of volume I of the third edition of the *International Pharmacopoeia* was sent for final comments to all WHO Member States, to members of the WHO Expert Advisory Panel on the International Pharmacopoeia and Pharmaceutical Preparations, and to other specialists.

The following specialists participated both in person and by correspondence in the above-mentioned discussions, and commented on the final draft: Professor E.A. Babayan, Ministry of Health, Moscow, USSR; Dr D. Banes, The United States Pharmacopoeia, Rockville, MD, USA; Dr. I. Bayer, National Institute of Pharmacy, Budapest, Hungary; Dr T. Bićan, Institute for the Control of Drugs, Zagreb, Yugoslavia; Mr J.Y. Binka, Government Chemical Laboratory, Accra, Ghana; Professor W.H. Briner, Duke University Medical Center, Durham, NC, USA; Mr J.R. Buriánek, State Institute for the Control of Drugs, Prague, Czechoslovakia; Dr T. Canbäck, Swedish Pharmacopoeia Commission, Stockholm, Sweden; Dr J.C. Charlton, The Radiochemical Centre, Amersham, England; Professor Y. Cohen, Atomic Energy Commission, Saclay, Gif-sur-Yvette, France; Dr D. Cook, Drug Research Laboratories, Ottawa, Ontario, Canada; Dr N. Diding, WHO Collaborating Centre for Chemical Reference Substances, Solna, Sweden; Dr L.F. Dodson, National Biological Standards Laboratory, Department of Health, Canberra, Australia; Dr K. Florey, The Squibb Institute for Medical Research, New Brunswick, NJ, USA; Ms M.A. Garth, National Center for Antibiotics Analysis, Food and Drug Administration, Washington, DC, USA; Dr A.R. Gennaro, The Philadelphia College of Pharmacy and Science, Philadelphia, PA, USA; Dr T. George, Ciba-Geigy Research Centre, Goregaon, Bombay, India; Mr W. Hewitt, Cheltenham, England; Mr Kang Hu, Peking Institute for the Control of Pharmaceutical and Biological Products, Peking, People's Republic of China; Dr T. Inoue, National Institute of Hygienic Sciences, Tokyo, Japan; Miss S. Johansson, WHO Collaborating Centre for Chemical Reference Substances, Solna, Sweden; Mr C.A. Johnson, British Pharmacopoeia Commission, London, England; Mr H.G. Kristensen, The Danish Pharmacopoeia Council, Brønshøj, Denmark; Dr K. Kristensen, The Isotope Pharmacy, Brønshøj, Denmark; Dr C.S. Kumkumian, Bureau of Drugs, Food and Drug Administration, Rockville, MD, USA; Dr E. Lang, Ciba-Geigy SA, Basle, Switzerland; Professor J. Laszlovszky, National Institute of Pharmacy, Budapest, Hungary; Dr T. Layloff, National Center for Drug Analysis, Food and Drug Administration, St Louis,

MO, USA; Dr J.W. Lightbown, National Institute for Biological Standards and Control, London, England; Dr A.J. Liston, Drugs Directorate, Ottawa, Ontario, Canada; Mr W.J. Mader, Alza Corporation, Palo Alto, CA, USA; Professor M.D. Maškovskij, Pharmacopoeia Committee of the USSR, Moscow, USSR; Dr E. Nieminen, Lääkelaboratorio, Helsinki, Finland; Dr A.N. Obojmakova, Pharmacopoeia Committee of the USSR, Moscow, USSR; Mr B. Öhrner, WHO Collaborating Centre for Chemical Reference Substances, Solna, Sweden; Dr T. Olawuyi Oke, Federal Drug Quality Control Laboratory, Yaba, Lagos State, Nigeria; Professor X. Perlia, Institut de Pharmacie, Zurich, Switzerland; Dr M. Pesez, Roussel Uclaf SA, Romainville, France; Professor J. Richter, Institut für Arzneimittelwesen der DDR, Berlin-Weissensee, German Democratic Republic; Dr G. Schwartzman, Bureau of Drugs, Food and Drug Administration, Washington, DC, USA; Professor S.D. Sokolov, All-Union Chemico-Pharmaceutical Research Institute, Moscow, USSR; Dr I. Suzuki, National Institute of Hygienic Sciences, Tokyo, Japan; Mr Tien Sung-chiu, Peking Institute for the Control of Pharmaceutical and Biological Products, Peking, People's Republic of China; Mr Tu Kuo-shih, Peking Institute for the Control of Phamaceutical and Biological Products, Peking, People's Republic of China; Dr M.M. Tuckerman, School of Pharmacy, Temple University, Philadelphia, PA, USA; Professor H. Vanderhaeghe, Rega Pharmaceutical Institute, Leuven, Belgium; Dr R. Vasiliev, State Institute for Drug Control and Pharmaceutical Research, Bucharest, Romania; Dr A. Végh, Hungarian Pharmacopoeia Commission, Budapest, Hungary; Mr W.J. Welsh, Radiation Medicine Division, Ottawa, Ontario, Canada; Dr B.A. Wills, Allen & Hanburys Ltd., Ware, England; Dr W.W. Wright, Bureau of Drugs, Food and Drug Administration, Washington, DC, USA.

Furthermore, comments were obtained from the International Atomic Energy Agency, the Austrian Pharmacopoeia Commission, the Danish Pharmacopoeia Council, the French National Pharmacopoeia Commission, the Pharmacopoeia Commission of the Federal Republic of Germany, the Hungarian Pharmacopoeia Commission, and the United States Pharmacopoeia; from the Ministries of Health of Bulgaria, Romania and Sweden; and also from the National Biological Standards Laboratory, Canberra, Australia, the Drug Research Laboratories, Ottawa, Ontario, Canada, and the Department of Scientific and Industrial Research, Wellington, New Zealand. In addition, some professional associations provided comments and suggestions.

The World Health Organization takes this opportunity to express its gratitude to all those persons and institutions who took part in the preparation of this volume.

Mr C.A. Johnson served as Chairman at the above-mentioned meetings of the WHO Expert Committee on Specifications for Pharmaceutical

Preparations. The functions of Secretary to the Committee were assumed by Mr O. Wallén, Chief Pharmaceutical Officer, WHO, and by Dr W. Wieniawski, Senior Pharmaceutical Officer, assisted by Miss M. Schmid, Technical Assistant.

Volume 1 of the third edition of the *International Pharmacopoeia* contains the description of 42 general methods of analysis. For most of the physical and physicochemical methods an introductory description is given followed by recommended procedures. This general description is designed to facilitate the utilization of these methods for the purpose of drug quality assurance, even outside the scope of specifications published in the *International Pharmacopoeia.*

In accordance with resolution WHA30.39[1] of the Thirtieth World Health Assembly the units of measurement used in the third edition of the *International Pharmacopoeia* are based on the International System of Units (SI) (see page 13).

The general notices that precede volume I of the third edition concern primarily terms and provisions applicable in connexion with the general methods of analysis and will be expanded in subsequent volumes.

In accordance with World Health Assembly resolution WHA3.10 mentioned above, the *International Pharmacopoeia* constitutes a collection of recommended methods and specifications that are not intended to have a legal status as such in any country, unless expressly introduced for that purpose by appropriate legislation, but are offered to serve as references so that national requirements can be established on a similar basis in any country. Any Member State of the World Health Organization may include all or part of these provisions in its national requirements.

All comments and suggestions concerning the contents of the *International Pharmacopoeia* will be examined, and suggested amendments considered for inclusion in subsequent volumes of the *International Pharmacopoeia.*

GENERAL NOTICES

Quantities and their precision

The quantities of substances and reagents to be used in the tests, assays, and procedures have to be measured with adequate precision. The required precision is indicated by the number of decimals given in the text. For example, 20 indicates a value not less than 19.5 and not greater

---

[1] *WHO Handbook of Resolutions and Decisions, vol. II, third edition, 1979, p. 99.*

than 20.5; 2.0 indicates a value not less than 1.95 and not greater than 2.05; and 0.20 a value not less than 0.195 and not greater than 0.205.

Temperature measurements and their precision

The required precision of temperature measurements is indicated in a manner similar to that given for the quantities of substance.

pH values and their precision

The required precision of pH values is indicated in a manner similar to that given for the quantities of substance.

Calculation of results

The results of assays should be calculated to one decimal place more than indicated in the requirement and then rounded up or down as follows: if the last figure calculated is 5 to 9, the preceding figure is increased by 1; if it is 4 or less, the preceding figure is left unchanged. Other calculations, for example, in the standardization of volumetric solutions, are carried out similarly.

Solutions

Unless otherwise specified, all solutions indicated in the tests and assays are prepared with distilled or demineralized water.

Solubility

Statements about the solubility of a substance refer to the approximate solubility at 20 °C, unless otherwise indicated. The expression "part" has to be understood as describing the number of millilitres of the solvent, represented by the stated number of parts, in which 1 g of the solid is soluble.

Descriptive terms are sometimes used to indicate the solubility of a substance. The following table indicates the meaning of such terms:

Descriptive term	Number of millilitres of the solvent required for 1 g of the solid
Very soluble	Less than 1
Freely soluble	From 1 to 10
Soluble	From 10 to 30
Sparingly soluble	From 30 to 100
Slightly soluble	From 100 to 1 000
Very slightly soluble	From 1 000 to 10 000
Practically insoluble	More than 10 000

Loss on drying

In determining the loss on drying, unless another amount of substance is specified, 1.0 g is dried under the conditions indicated.

Constant weight

The expression "dry to constant weight" means that the drying process should be continued until the results of two consecutive weighings do not differ by more than 0.5 mg per g of the substance taken for the determination, the second weighing being made after an additional hour of drying at the prescribed conditions. The expression "ignite to constant weight" has a similar meaning, the second weighing following further ignition.

Containers

The container and its closure must not interact physically or chemically with the substance it holds so as to alter its purity or strength. The following terms describe additional requirements for the permeability of containers:

Well-closed container. It must protect the contents from extraneous matter or from loss of the substance under ordinary or customary conditions of handling, shipment, or storage.

Tightly closed container. It must protect the contents from extraneous matter, from loss of the substance, and from efflorescence, deliquescence, or evaporation under ordinary or customary conditions of handling, shipment, or storage, and shall be capable of tight reclosure.

Protection from light

The substance required to be kept protected from light should be maintained in a light-resistant container that shields the contents against the effects of light, either by reason of the inherent properties of the material from which the container is composed, or because a special coating has been applied to the container. Alternatively, the container may be placed inside a suitable light-resistant (opaque) covering.

Patents and trademarks

The inclusion in the *International Pharmacopoeia* of any product subject to actual, or potential, patent or similar rights, or the inclusion of any name that is a trademark in any part of the world, does not and shall not be deemed to imply or convey permission, authority, or licence to exercise any right or privilege protected by such patent or trademark, including licence to manufacture, without due permission, authority, or licence from the person or persons in whom such rights and privileges are vested.

Use of trade names

Reference to a particular trade name in the description of certain materials used in assays and tests does not imply that other, equivalent, materials are not also suitable.

Reagents, test solutions and volumetric solutions

The letters R, IR, TS and VS following the names of reagents, test solutions and volumetric solutions indicate that they are described in the list commencing on p. 167.

UNITS OF MEASUREMENT

The names and symbols for units of measurement used by the *International Pharmacopoeia* are those of the *Système international d'Unités* (International System of Units) (SI), a practical system of units that has been developed through the efforts of the General Conference of Weights and Measures (CGPM) and other international organizations. The 11th General Conference (1960) adopted the international abbreviation SI for this system of units[1].

The SI units used in the third edition of the *International Pharmacopoeia*, as well as their multiples and submultiples, are in many cases identical to the units used for the respective units of measurement in the second edition. In other cases, however, the SI has introduced differently defined units; this is especially true for derived units. In such situations, to promote better understanding of the procedures and limits related to quality requirements, the third edition of the *International Pharmacopoeia* gives, in addition to the SI units, the units previously used in the second edition, together with appropriate conversion of numerical values.

---

[1] Complete information on SI units is contained in *A guide to international recommendations on names and symbols for quantities and on units of measurement*, by D.A. Lowe, Geneva, World Health Organization, 1975; a more concise account is given in *The SI for the health professions*, Geneva, World Health Organization, 1977.

The following multiplicative prefixes, which indicate decimal multiples and submultiples of the SI units, are used in the *International Pharmacopoeia:*

giga   (G) 10^9
mega (M) 10^6
kilo   (k) 10^3
centi (c) 10^{-2}
milli (m) 10^{-3}
micro (μ) 10^{-6}
nano (n) 10^{-9}
pico   (p) 10^{-12}

The use of these prefixes is illustrated by the following units, multiples and submultiples, that are employed in the third edition of the *International Pharmacopoeia:*

Units of length
metre   (m)
centimetre   (cm)
millimetre   (mm)
micrometre (μm)
nanometre   (nm)

Units of volume (capacity)
litre   (l) $= 1\ 000\ cm^3$
millilitre   (ml) $= 1\ cm^3$
microlitre   (μl) $= 0.001\ cm^3$

Units of temperature
Kelvin   (K)
degree Celsius   (^{0}C)

Units of mass
kilogram   (kg)
gram   (g)
milligram   (mg)
microgram   (μg)
nanogram   (ng)

Units of time
year   (a)
day   (d)
hour   (h)
minute   (min)
second   (s)
millisecond   (ms)
microsecond (μs)

Units of pressure
kilopascal   (kPa)
pascal   (Pa)

The following non-SI units of pressure are also used in some special cases:

pound-force per square inch (lbf/in^2 or,
incorrectly, psi) $\approx$ 0.69 kPa
millimetre of mercury (mmHg) $\approx$ 133 Pa

Units of radioactivity [1]
gigabecquerel (GBq) = 27.03 mCi
megabecquerel (MBq) = 27.03 μCi
becquerel   (Bq)   = 27.03 pCi
curie   (Ci)   = 37 GBq
millicurie   (mCi) = 37 MBq
microcurie   (μCi) = 37 kBq

Units of electric current
ampere   (A)
milliampere (mA)
nanoampere (nA)

Units of electric potential
volt   (V)
millivolt   (mV)

Unit of resistance
ohm   (Ω)

---

[1] The definition of units of radioactivity is given under "Radiopharmaceuticals" (see pages 52-55).

PHYSICAL METHODS

MEASUREMENT OF MASS

Tests that involve the measurement of mass require the use of balances of capacity and sensitivity corresponding to the degree of accuracy sought.

When weighing quantities of 50 mg or more that are to be "accurately weighed", an analytical balance of 100-200 g capacity and 0.1 mg sensitivity is required. When weighing quantities of less than 50 mg that are to be "accurately weighed", an analytical balance of 20 g capacity and 0.001 mg sensitivity, usually called an analytical microbalance, is required.

Balances of lower sensitivity are used for other tests in which a measurement of mass is involved.

Apparatus

Analytical balances should possess adequate capacity and sensitivity. They may be either of the equal-arm type, requiring the use of a set of calibrated weights, or of any other suitable type (for example, analytical microbalances using magnetic measurement) provided that their performance is periodically checked by means of a reference set of calibrated weights.

The analytical balance should be so constructed as to support its full capacity without developing undue stress and its sensitivity should not be altered by repeated weighings of the full-capacity load. It should preferably be equipped with a damping device (for example, a magnetic or air damper) that causes the beam to come quickly to rest (aperiodic balance).

The analytical balance may be constructed for manual placement of all weights or, preferably, be equipped with a weight-loading device for the whole or part of the balance range. In the latter case it should be equipped with loading registers clearly indicating the load applied. Furthermore, the analytical balance may be equipped with an optical scale projection system, usually encompassing a part of the balance range (e.g., where the displacement of the projected scale relative to the datum line gives a direct reading of weight), or a read-out device of any other type.

The type of analytical balance having constant sensitivity over the whole capacity range is the constant-load, single-pan balance. It has a set of weights suspended from a counterpoised beam; in the process of weighing, these are removed from the beam by a manually operated mechanical device until equilibrium is reached.

The analytical balance should be constructed in a proper housing with suitable openings to permit the placement of weighed material. The openings should be constructed in such a way as to exclude air currents. Desiccants may be placed inside the housing (e.g., silica gel, anhydrous calcium chloride) for the maintenance of a relatively dry atmosphere.

Sets of calibrated weights used with balances that require manual placement of weights and sets of weights used to check the sensitivity of balances of another type should be kept in a case made of suitable material and properly lined.

Placement of balance

The analytical balance should be placed upon a firm foundation that is as free from mechanical vibration as possible, preferably on an antivibration table of proper design. Alternatively, it may be placed on a concrete slab resting upon piers that are either sunk into the ground or connected to the construction elements of the building; or it may be placed upon a stout table or shelf protected by shock absorbers, such as cork mats or sheet rubber.

The balance should also be protected from humidity and acid fumes, preferably by placing it in a separate room of the laboratory. It should not be near a window or radiator, in direct sunlight, or in a position where draughts may come into contact with it.

The balance should be equipped with a levelling device and an indicator of proper position. Proper adjustment of levelling should be frequently checked.

Checking of sensitivity

The sensitivity of the balance should be periodically checked by a qualified expert.

RECOMMENDED PROCEDURE

Checking the stability of the equilibrium position

Before the balance is used, its equilibrium position without load should be checked several times. After each test, the balance has to be arrested.

The equilibrium position of the balance under load should also be determined from time to time, for example, with one-tenth of the full load and with the full load. The difference between equilibrium positions found in two successive determinations made with equal loads should not exceed 0.1 mg for analytical balances and 0.001 mg for analytical microbalances.

Operation of the balance

When the balance is not in use the balance beam and pan supports should be raised. The doors of the housing should always be kept closed.

To release the balance, the beam and pans should be lowered very carefully.

Objects to be weighed must be allowed to attain the temperature of the balance before weighing is started. The object to be weighed, as well as the weights, should always be placed on the pan as centrally as possible. During a weighing or on any occasion when objects are being added to or removed from the pans, both the beam arrests and the pan supports must be raised. Substances must be weighed in suitable containers such as beakers, weighing bottles, or crucibles. Liquids and volatile or hygroscopic solids must be weighed in tightly closed vessels, such as stoppered weighing bottles. No chemicals or objects that might injure the balance pans should be placed directly upon them.

When small quantities of a substance (for example, the sulfated ash) must be weighed in a large vessel and a fairly long period elapses between the two weighings, atmospheric pressure and temperature may alter sufficiently to affect the buoyancy and thus cause an appreciable error. In two-pan balances, this error may be eliminated by using another vessel of similar shape and weight for taring.

The pans of the balance should be periodically lightly brushed with a camel-hair or similar brush to remove any dust that may have collected.

The weights should be handled only by means of a pair of forceps, which should possess tips covered with suitable material.

DETERMINATION OF MELTING TEMPERATURE, MELTING RANGE, CONGEALING POINT, BOILING POINT, AND BOILING RANGE

The thermodynamically true melting point of a substance (the triple point) is a physical constant that is indicative of the identity and purity of the material. It is defined as the temperature at which the solid, liquid, and gaseous phases of the substance are in equilibrium in an evacuated, closed system. Under normal atmospheric pressure the solid and liquid phases of a substance are in equilibrium at a temperature that differs somewhat from the triple point but, since pressure effects on the solid-liquid transition temperature are minimal, this difference does not, in general, exceed a few hundredths of a degree Celsius.

Methods for the determination of equilibrium melting points are laborious and require complicated equipment. The usual practice is therefore to estimate melting points by dynamic rather than equilibrium methods. The melting points thus determined usually differ significantly from the corresponding triple points. The magnitude of the deviation varies with the particular method employed, with the criterion adopted as the "melting point", and possibly with the substance under examination. Melting points determined by the capillary method of the *International Pharmacopoeia* are typically about one degree higher than the thermodynamically true melting points.

Determination of melting points (called subsequently melting temperatures) is used in pharmacopoeial specifications primarily for identification of the substance concerned. The validity of the identification is greatly enhanced if the so-called mixed-melting point procedure is applied. This involves an additional determination to demonstrate that the substance being examined and a mixture prepared of equal parts of this substance and an authentic specimen (reference substance) of the substance melt at the same temperature. If the two substances are not identical the mixture normally melts at a significantly lower temperature than the substance being examined, and the melting range is relatively broad.

The presence of impurities in a substance results in a more or less pronounced lowering of its melting point. Even more significant is that impurities present in the substance may cause its melting range to be extended. In most cases where melting behaviour is used as a criterion of purity the *International Pharmacopoeia* therefore prescribes determination of the melting range rather than the melting point.

Similarly for liquids, determinations of boiling point and boiling range give information that contributes to the identification and purity estimation of liquid compounds. Practical considerations again dictate the use of methods that yield apparent constants that may differ from the thermodynamically true values. However, if the prescribed experimental conditions are closely adhered to, the results obtained are of sufficient reproducibility.

A. Determination of Melting Temperature and Melting Range of Pulverizable Substances

The *melting range* of a substance is the range between the corrected temperature at which the substance begins to collapse or form droplets on the wall of a capillary tube and the corrected temperature at which it is completely melted as shown by the disappearance of the solid phase.

The statement in a monograph "melting range $a–b$ °C" means that the melting range determined by the method below must fall within these limits.

The *melting temperature* of a substance is the corrected temperature at which it is completely melted as shown by the disappearance of the solid phase.

Apparatus

A suitable apparatus for the determination consists of a glass vessel with appropriate liquid, a controlled source of heat, a thermometer, a capillary tube, and a magnifying glass.

The glass vessel should have a suitable construction, contain an appropriate liquid and be fitted with a stirring device capable of rapid mixing of the liquid (certain liquid silicones are suitable). The controlled source of heat should be capable of raising the temperature of the liquid heating medium at the required rate.

Standardized thermometers should cover the range −10 to +360 °C, the length of one degree on the scale being not less than 0.8 mm. These thermometers should preferably be of the mercury-in-glass, solid-stem type with a cylindrical bulb and made of approved thermometric glass suitable for the range covered; each thermometer should have a safety chamber.

Thermometers used for determination of melting temperatures may be calibrated for total or partial immersion. A *total-immersion thermometer* should read correctly when it is immersed at least to the end of the liquid column in the medium the temperature of which is to be measured. A *partial-immersion thermometer* should read correctly when it is immersed to a prescribed depth, and when the emergent liquid column is under prescribed conditions. When total-immersion thermometers are used partially immersed, an auxiliary thermometer is required for the determination of the emergent-stem correction. These two thermometers should be surrounded with a glass tube above the surface of the heating material.

The capillary tube should be made of borosilicate glass, closed at one end, and have the following dimensions: thickness of the wall, about 0.10-0.15 mm; length, suitable for the apparatus used; internal diameter, 0.9-1.1 mm.

A suitable magnifying-glass should be used for observation of the capillary tube.

Other apparatus or methods may be used provided they are capable of equal accuracy and have been calibrated against the method of the *International Pharmacopoeia* by means of the WHO Melting Point Reference Substances[1].

---

[1] A set of substances with melting points according to the *International Pharmacopoeia* in the temperature range +69 to +263 ºC. The substances are available from the WHO Collaborating Centre for Chemical Reference Substances, Box 3045, S-171 03 Solna, Sweden.

RECOMMENDED PROCEDURE

Spread a small quantity of the finely powdered substance in a thin layer and dry it in a vacuum desiccator over silica gel, desiccant, R, phosphorus pentoxide R, or other suitable desiccant for 24 hours, or at a temperature specified in the monograph.

Transfer a quantity of the dried powder to a dry capillary tube and pack the powder, for example, by tapping the tube on a hard surface, so as to form a tightly packed column about 3 mm in height. Introduce the capillary tube into the heated bath at a temperature 5 °C below the expected lower limit of the melting range, the rise of temperature being regulated beforehand to 1 °C per minute, unless either the temperature of the introduction of the capillary tube into the bath or the rate of temperature rise are otherwise specified in the monograph. The capillary tube should be fitted in the bath in such a way that its closed end is at the level of the middle of the bulb of the standard thermometer.

When a thermometer calibrated for partial immersion is used, care must be taken that it is immersed exactly to its immersion mark when the readings are taken.

Unless otherwise specified in the monograph, readings are taken of the temperature at which the substance is observed to collapse or form droplets on the wall of the tube and of the temperature at which it is completely melted as indicated by the disappearance of the solid phase.

To the temperature readings add the correction for deviation of the standard thermometer. When thermometers calibrated for total immersion are used partially immersed, add to the readings of the standard thermometer also the emergent-stem correction, which is obtained as follows:

Before starting the determination of the melting range, an auxiliary thermometer is attached so that the bulb touches the standard thermometer at a point midway between the graduation for the expected melting point and the surface of the heating material. When the substance has melted the temperature is read on the auxiliary thermometer. The correction to be added to the temperature reading of the standard thermometer is calculated from the following formula:

$$0.00015 \ N(T{-}t)$$

where T is the temperature reading of the standard thermometer;

t is the temperature reading of the auxiliary thermometer;

N is the number of degrees of the scale of the standard thermometer between the surface of the heating material and the level of the mercury.

When needed, the emergent-stem correction for thermometers calibrated for partial immersion may be calculated from the same formula as above, but replacing T by T_s, which is the mean temperature of the emergent-stem of the thermometer at the time of calibration.

Both the above-mentioned corrections for emergent-stem and any deviation of the standard thermometer may conveniently be replaced by calibration of the apparatus by means of the WHO Melting Point Reference Substances.

B. Determination of Melting Point of Fats, Waxes, etc.

The melting point of fats, waxes, etc. is the corrected temperature at which the column of substance in the capillary tube becomes transparent or moves upwards, when tested by the method described below.

Apparatus

A similar apparatus to that described under A for the determination of melting temperature and melting range of pulverizable substances should be used with the following modifications:

— water should be used in the heating vessel;
— an accurately standardized thermometer should cover the range —10 to +100 °C;
— a glass capillary tube should have the same dimensions as described under A but be open at both ends; soft glass capillary tubes may be used.

RECOMMENDED PROCEDURE

Unless otherwise specified in the monograph, melt the substance at as low a temperature as possible, and then suck the liquid up to a height of about 10 mm in the capillary tube. Cool the charged tube at 10 °C or lower for 24 hours. If the monograph specifies that the melting temperature is to be determined without previous melting of the substance, charge the capillary tube by pushing it into the unmelted substance so that a column about 10 mm long is forced in. The determination may then be carried out immediately. Attach the tube to the thermometer in the water-bath by means of a rubber band or otherwise so that the lower end of the capillary tube is at the level of the middle of the bulb of the thermometer, and the distance between the lower end of the capillary tube and the water level is about 20 mm. Heat the bath with constant stirring, the heating being regulated so that the temperature rise, at a temperature of 5 °C below the expected melting temperature, is about 1 °C per minute.

C. Determination of Congealing Point

The congealing point of a liquid or of a melted solid is the highest temperature at which it solidifies. The congealing point of the liquid is the same as the melting temperature of the solid, but since the liquid may be cooled to a temperature below its congealing point without assuming the solid form, the method described below is used to determine the congealing point of a liquid or of a melted solid.

Apparatus

A suitable apparatus consists of a test-tube of about 2 cm internal diameter and about 10 cm in length, suspended by means of a bored cork inside a larger tube, about 3 cm in diameter and 12 cm in length, a vessel with water or suitable freezing mixture, and an accurately standardized thermometer.

RECOMMENDED PROCEDURE

Unless otherwise specified in the monograph, place in the inner test-tube about 10 ml of the liquid, or 10 g of the melted solid, to be tested and cool together the inner and the outer tubes in water or in a suitable freezing mixture to a temperature about 5 °C below the expected congealing point of the liquid; with the thermometer gently stir the liquid until it begins to solidify. At first there is a gradual fall in temperature. Then, as the solid phase forms, the temperature remains constant for some time or rises before becoming constant. The highest temperature observed is regarded as the congealing point. If the liquid does not start to congeal within 2 °C of the expected temperature, congelation may be induced by adding a small crystal of the substance to the liquid or by rubbing the inner walls of the test-tube with the thermometer.

D. Determination of Boiling Point

The boiling point of a liquid is the corrected temperature at which the liquid boils under normal atmospheric pressure when determined by the method described below.

Apparatus

A suitable apparatus for the determination consists of a vessel with appropriate liquid, a source of heat, and a thermometer, as described under A for the determination of melting temperature and melting range for pulverizable substances; also needed are a thin-walled test-tube of glass of external diameter about 4 mm and length suitable for the apparatus used and a thin-walled capillary tube of glass of internal diameter not exceeding 1 mm, which should be closed by fusing about 2 mm from one end.

RECOMMENDED PROCEDURE

Transfer 3-4 drops of the liquid to be tested (or the equivalent quantity of a solid compound) to the test-tube. Place the capillary tube (fused end down) in the test-tube and introduce the test-tube into the heating bath in such a way that its lower end is at the level of the middle of the bulb of the thermometer. Heat the bath rapidly with constant stirring to a temperature about 10 °C below the expected boiling point, then regulate the heating so that the temperature rise is 1–2 °C per minute. During the heating bubbles begin to escape from the lower end of the capillary tube, slowly at first but then more rapidly as the temperature approaches the boiling point. Read the temperature at which bubbles are released in an even rapid stream and then decrease the heating so that the temperature of the bath falls 1–2 °C per minute. Read the temperature at which the release of bubbles ceases. The boiling point is taken as the average of the two temperatures, corrections for emergent-stem of the thermometer and for deviation from normal atmospheric pressure being applied as necessary. Obtain the emergent-stem correction as described under A for the determination of melting temperature and melting range of pulverizable substances. If the determination is made at a barometric pressure that deviates from 101.3 kPa (760 mmHg), add to the temperatures the following correction:

$$k(p - p_1)$$

where p is the standard barometric pressure;

p_1 is the barometric pressure read on a mercury barometer, without taking into account the temperature of the air; and

k is the boiling temperature increment, as indicated below.

For pressures read on a barometer calibrated in kPa, use the following data:

$p = 101.3$

$k = 0.3$ (boiling temperature increment produced by a rise of pressure of 1 kPa), unless otherwise specified in the monograph.

For pressures read on a barometer calibrated in mmHg, use the following data:

$p = 760$

$k = 0.04$ (boiling temperature increment produced by a rise of pressure of 1 mmHg), unless otherwise specified in the monograph.

E. Determination of Boiling Range (Distillation Range)

The boiling range (distillation range) is the corrected range of temperature, within which the whole or a specified portion of a liquid distils, under normal atmospheric pressure, when determined by the method described below.

Apparatus

A suitable apparatus for the determination consists of a distillation flask, a condenser, a receiver, a heat source with heat shields, and a thermometer.

The distillation flask of 50–60 ml capacity is made of heat-resistant glass. Flasks with the following dimensions are suitable: neck 10–12 cm long and 14–16 mm in internal diameter with a side-arm, 10–12 cm long and about 5 mm in internal diameter, attached at about the midway point of the neck and forming an angle of 70–75° with the lower portion of the neck.

The condenser is either a straight glass condenser, made of heat-resistant glass, 55–60 cm in length with a water jacket about 40 cm in length, or a condenser of another design having equivalent condensing capacity. The lower end of the condenser may be bent to provide a delivery tube, or a bent adapter may be attached to it to serve as a delivery tube.

The receiver consists of a 25–50-ml measuring cylinder graduated in subdivisions of 0.5 ml.

The heat source consists of a small gas burner, preferably of a Bunsen type, or an electric heater or mantle capable of adjustment comparable to that possible with the gas burner. If a gas burner is used, an asbestos shield is placed around the flask near its bottom. The shield is made of asbestos board, 5–7 mm thick, in the form of a square with sides of 14–16 cm and with a perforation in the centre. The diameter of the latter should be such that when the flask is set into it, the portion of the flask below the upper surface of the asbestos board has a capacity of 3–4 ml.

The thermometer should preferably be calibrated for partial immersion of 100 mm as described under A for the determination of melting temperature and melting range of pulverizable substances; otherwise a total-immersion thermometer may be used with appropriate emergent-stem correction. When the thermometer is placed in position, the stem should be located in the centre of the neck of the flask, and the top of the bulb should be just below the bottom of the outlet to the side-arm.

RECOMMENDED PROCEDURE

Place in the flask 25 ml of the liquid to be tested, taking care not to allow any of the liquid to enter the side-arm, and add 0.3–0.5 g of glass-beads or other suitable substance. Shield the burner and the flask from external air currents and apply heat so that the vapour rises only slowly into the neck of the flask and between 5–10 minutes elapse before the first drop of distillate falls from the condenser. Continue the distillation at the rate of 2–3 ml per minute, collecting the distillate in the receiver. Read the temperature when the first drop of distillate falls from the condenser, and again when the last quantity of liquid evaporates from the bottom of the flask or when the specified percentage has distilled over.

The boiling ranges (distillation ranges) indicated in the monographs are applied at a barometric pressure of 101.3 kPa (760 mmHg). If the determination is made at some other barometric pressure, correct the observed temperature readings for any difference in the barometric pressure by allowing 0.1 °C for each 0.36 kPa (2.7 mmHg) of the difference, adding if the pressure is lower, or subtracting if the pressure is higher.

DETERMINATION OF MASS DENSITY
AND RELATIVE DENSITY

The mass density (ϱ) of a substance is the mass of one unit volume of the substance. In terms of SI base units, mass density is expressed in kilograms per cubic metre. However, in the *International Pharmacopoeia* the mass density is expressed in kilograms per litre (which is equivalent to grams per millilitre) at a temperature of 20 °C (ϱ_{20}) and it is corrected for buoyancy (i.e., reduced to vacuum conditions). For pharmacopoeial purposes the mass density of liquids is not measured directly but calculated from their relative density.

The relative density d_{20}^{20} is the ratio of the mass of the substance in air at 20 °C to that of an equal volume of water at the same temperature. The term "relative density d_{20}^{20}" is equivalent to the formerly used term "specific gravity determined at 20 °C".

The relative density d_4^{20} denotes the ratio of the mass of the substance in air at 20 °C to that of an equal volume of water at 4 °C. As the relative density of water at 20 °C is 0.998234, these values are related by the following equation:

$$d_4^{20} = 0.998234 \, d_{20}^{20}.$$

RECOMMENDED PROCEDURE

Determine the relative density (d_{20}^{20}) using a hydrostatic balance (only when the precision indicated in the monograph is three decimal digits) or a pycnometer.

If the value of mass density ϱ_{20} (in kg/l or g/ml) is referred to in the monograph, carry out the measurement of relative density and from the value obtained calculate the mass density according to the formula:

$$\varrho_{20} = 0.99703 \, d_{20}^{20} + 0.0012.$$

Use of a hydrostatic balance

Use an instrument of suitable construction placed on a horizontal support. The plummet (diver) should be suspended on a thin wire, made preferably of platinum. To calibrate the instrument equilibrate the plummet in the air, then immerse it in the cylinder filled with water and equilibrate again by placing suitable riders (weights) at appropriate notches along the beam. The plummet should swim freely in the liquid. Fill the cylinder with the test liquid and carry out the measurement in a similar way. Take care that the length of the immersed portion of the suspending wire is similar in all measurements. The weight that has to be added to obtain the equilibrium in the test liquid (or to be subtracted in the case of liquids of density lower than that of water) gives directly the measure of its relative density.

Use of a pycnometer

Use a pycnometer of suitable form of a capacity of not less than 5 ml. Weigh accurately the empty, dry pycnometer, and fill it with the test liquid brought previously to a temperature of about 20 °C. Hold the filled pycnometer at a temperature of 20 ± 1 °C for about 30 minutes, adjust the liquid to the mark using, if necessary, a small strip of filter-paper to remove the excess and to wipe the inlet from the inside, and weigh accurately. Calculate the weight of the liquid in the pycnometer. Remove the liquid, clean and dry the pycnometer, repeat the measurement with carbon-dioxide-free water R, also at 20 ± 1 °C, and calculate the weight of water in the pycnometer. The ratio of the weights of the test liquid and of water gives the relative density (d_{20}^{20}).

DETERMINATION OF OPTICAL ROTATION
AND SPECIFIC ROTATION

Many substances possess the inherent property to rotate the plane of incident polarized light; this property is called optical activity. The measurement of optical activity is used for pharmacopoeial purposes mainly to establish the identity of the substance. It may also be employed to test the purity of the substance (absence of optically non-active foreign substances) and as an assay procedure.

Optical rotation

The optical rotation is the angle through which the plane of polarization is rotated when polarized light passes through a layer of a liquid. Substances are described as dextrorotatory or levorotatory according to whether the plane of polarization is rotated clockwise or counterclockwise, respectively, as determined by viewing towards the light source. Dextrorotation is designated (+) and levorotation is designated (−).

In the *International Pharmacopoeia* the optical rotation (α) is expressed in angular degrees. In the SI, the angle of optical rotation is expressed in radians (rad).

The optical rotation is measured on a layer of suitable thickness at the wavelength specified in the monograph. If the sodium D line is specified, the sodium light of wavelength 589.3 nm (a mean value for a doublet at 589.0 nm and 589.6 nm) should be used. The wavelength of the mercury green line at 546.1 nm is also frequently used. If the wavelength specified lies in the ultraviolet range, the use of a photoelectric polarimeter is necessary.

The measurement of optical rotation should be carried out at the temperature indicated in the monograph, usually at 20–25 °C. Some substances have large temperature coefficients and for them special care should be taken to adjust the temperature indicated.

Specific optical rotation (specific rotation)

The specific optical rotation of a liquid substance is the angle of rotation measured as specified in the monograph, calculated with reference to a layer 100 mm thick, and divided by the relative density (specific gravity) measured at the temperature at which the rotation is measured.

The specific optical rotation of a solid is the angle of rotation measured as specified in the monograph, and calculated with reference to a layer 100 mm thick of a solution containing 1 g of the substance per ml.

$$\text{Specific rotation} = \frac{10\,000a}{lc} = \frac{10\,000a}{ldp}$$

where a is the observed rotation, l is the length of the observed layer in mm, c is the number of g of substance contained in 100 ml of solution, d is the relative density and p is the number of g of substance contained in 100 g of solution.

In the *International Pharmacopoeia* the specific optical rotation is expressed as $[a]_\lambda^t$ where t is the temperature and λ the wavelength. For solid substances the solvent, if different from water, and the concentration are further described. The general directions concerning wavelength and temperature as given above for optical rotation refer equally to the measurement of specific optical rotation. In the SI specific optical rotation (optical rotatory power) is given in $m^2\cdot rad/kg$ and molar optical rotatory power (a_n) in $m^2\cdot rad/mol$.

Apparatus

Optical rotation is measured with a polarimeter. The zero point of the polarimeter is determined with the tube empty but closed for liquid substances and filled with the specified solvent for solutions of solid substances.

Generally, a polarimeter accurate to 0.05° of angular rotation, and capable of being read with the same precision, suffices for pharmacopoeial purposes; in some cases, a polarimeter accurate to 0.01° of angular rotation, and read with comparable precision, may be required.

Polarimeters for visual measurement: commercial instruments are normally constructed for use with sodium light or a mercury-vapour lamp. The manufacturer's instructions relating to a suitable light source should be followed.

Photoelectric polarimeters: where it is directed in the individual monograph to determine the optical rotation photoelectrically, use a photoelectric polarimeter capable of an accuracy of at least 0.01°.

Measurement of optical rotation

The accuracy and precision of optical rotatory measurements will be increased if they are carried out with due regard for the following general considerations.

Optical elements of the instrument must be brilliantly clean and in exact alignment. The match point should lie close to the normal zero mark. The light source should be rigidly set and well aligned with respect to the optical bench. It should be supplemented by a filtering system capable of transmitting light of a sufficiently monochromatic nature. Precision polarimeters are generally designed to accommodate interchangeable discs to isolate the D line from sodium light or the 546.1 nm line efrom the mercury spectrum. With polarimeters not thus designed, cells containing suitably coloured liquids may be employed as filters.

Observations should be accurate and reproducible to the extent that differences between replicates, or between observed and true values of rotation (the latter value having been established by calibration of the polarimeter scale with suitable standards), shall not exceed one-fourth of the range given in the individual monograph for the rotation of the substance being tested.

Polarimeter tubes should be filled in such a way as to avoid creating or leaving air bubbles, which interfere with the passage of the beam of light. Interference from bubbles is minimized by the use of tubes in which the bore is expanded at one end. However, with tubes of uniform bore, such as semi-micro or micro tubes, care is required for proper filling.

In closing tubes having removable end-plates fitted with gaskets and caps, the latter should be tightened only enough to ensure a leak-proof seal between the end-plate and the body of the tube. Excessive pressure on the end-plate may set up strains that result in interference with the measurement. In determining the optical rotation of a substance of low rotatory power, it is desirable to loosen the caps and tighten them again between successive readings in the measurement of both the rotation and the zero point. In this way, differences arising from end-plate strain will generally be revealed and appropriate adjustments to eliminate the cause can be made.

The requirements for optical rotation and specific rotation apply to the dried, anhydrous, or solvent-free material in all those monographs in which standards for loss on drying, water, or solvent content are given. In calculating the result, the loss on drying, water, or solvent content determined by the method specified in the monograph should be taken into account.

RECOMMENDED PROCEDURE

If the substance is a solid, weigh a suitable portion and transfer it to a volumetric flask by means of water, or other solvent if specified in the monograph, reserving a portion of the solvent for the blank determination. Add enough solvent to bring the meniscus close to, but still below, the mark, and adjust the temperature of the flask contents by suspending the flask in a constant-temperature bath. Add solvent to the mark, and mix. Transfer the solution to the polarimeter tube, preferably within 30 minutes from the time the substance was dissolved, taking care to standardize the elapsed time in the case of substances known to undergo racemization or mutarotation. During the elapsed time interval, maintain the solution at the required temperature.

If the substance is a liquid, adjust its temperature, if necessary, and transfer it directly to the polarimeter tube.

When a polarimeter is used for visual measurement, make at least 6 readings of the observed rotation at the required temperature. Take half the readings in a clockwise and the other half in a counterclockwise direction. Substitute the reserved solvent for the solution, and make an equal number of readings on it. In the case of liquid substances, carry out blank determinations on the empty, dry tube. The zero correction is the average of the blank readings, and is subtracted from the average observed rotation if the two figures are of the same sign, or added if they are opposite in sign, to give the corrected observed rotation.

When a photoelectric polarimeter is used, a smaller number of readings is required, depending on the type of instrument.

DETERMINATON OF REFRACTIVE INDEX

The refractive index (n) of a substance is the ratio of the velocity of light in a vacuum to its velocity in the substance. It varies with the wavelength of the light used in its measurement and with the temperature. It is therefore necessary to specify these conditions (n_D^t). In practice it is usually convenient to measure the refraction with respect to air and the substance, rather than with respect to a vacuum and the substance, since, for pharmacopoeial purposes, this has no significant influence on the observed values.

The refractive index may also be defined as the ratio of the sine of the angle of incidence to the sine of the angle of refraction.

The measurement of the refractive index is employed for pharmacopoeial purposes mainly to establish the identity of liquid substances. It may also be used to test the purity of such substances.

Refractive indices are usually stated in terms of sodium light of wavelength 589.3 nm (line D) at a temperature of $20 \pm 0.5\ °C$ (n_D^{20}).

The accuracy of the measurement should be related to the requirements of the monograph. For pharmacopoeial purposes it is usually adequate to express the refractive index to three decimal places.

Apparatus

Commercial refractometers are normally constructed for use with white light but are calibrated to give the refractive index in terms of the sodium light of wavelength 589.3 nm (line D).

The optical parts of the apparatus should be kept brilliantly clean. The working surfaces of prisms should be free from scratches.

Subject to the directions given above, the manufacturer's instructions relating to a suitable light source should be followed.

The instrument should be calibrated against a standard provided by the manufacturer; the temperature control of the liquid being examined and the cleanliness of the prism should be checked frequently by determining the refractive index of distilled water, which is 1.3330 at 20 °C and 1.3325 at 25 °C.

SPECTROPHOTOMETRY IN THE VISIBLE AND ULTRAVIOLET REGIONS

Absorption spectrophotometry is the measurement of the absorption, by substances, of electromagnetic radiation of definite and narrow wavelength range, essentially monochromatic.

The spectral range used in the measurements described below extends from the short wavelengths of the ultraviolet through the visible region of the spectrum. For convenience of reference, this range may be regarded as consisting of two regions, the ultraviolet (190–380 nm) and the visible (380–780 nm).

Spectrophotometry in the visible region (formerly the term colorimetry was commonly used) is the measurement of absorption of visible light, which is usually not monochromatic but restricted by the use of pigmented or interference filters.

The ultraviolet and visible spectra of a substance generally do not have a high degree of specificity. Nevertheless, they are highly suitable for quantitative assay, and for many substances they are useful as additional means of identification.

General agreement has not yet been reached on the definition of terms used in spectrophotometry. The terms in italics used in connexion with spectrophotometric tests in the *International Pharmacopoeia* are defined as follows:

Absorbance (A) — The logarithm, to the base 10, of the reciprocal of the transmittance (*T*). The term internal transmission density may be used as a synonym of absorbance; descriptive terms formerly used included optical density, absorbancy, and extinction.

Transmittance (T) — The ratio of the radiant flux transmitted by the test substance to that of the incident radiant flux. Terms formerly used include transmittancy and transmission.

Absorptivity (a) — The quotient of the absorbance (A) divided by the product of the concentration of the substance (c), expressed in g per litre, and the absorption path length (b) expressed in cm ($a = A/bc$). Two terms closely related to absorptivity are specific extinction and specific absorption coefficient. The term "specific extinction" ($E_{1\ cm}^{1\ \%}$), as generally used in pharmacopoeias, denotes the quotient of the absorbance (A) divided by the product of the concentration of the substance (c), expressed in g per 100 ml, and the absorption path length (b) expressed in cm; therefore $E_{1\ cm}^{1\ \%} = 10a$. The term "specific absorption coefficient", tentatively proposed by the Commission on Physicochemical Symbols, Terminology and Units of the International Union of Pure and Applied Chemistry (IUPAC), is defined as the quotient of absorbance (A) divided by the product of concentration (c) and the absorption path length (l); when the symbol a_{SI} is utilized for specific absorption coefficient, which in the SI should be expressed in m^2 per kg, $a_{SI} = 100a$. The term " absorptivity " is not to be confused with absorbancy index or extinction coefficient.

Molar absorptivity (ε) — The quotient of the absorbance (A) divided by the product of the concentration of the substance (c), expressed in moles per litre, and the absorption path length (b) in cm. It is also the product of the absorptivity (a) and the molecular weight of the substance. The term molar absorption coefficient (linear) recommended by the Commission on Physicochemical Symbols, Terminology and Units of IUPAC is defined as the quotient of the internal transmission density (absorbance) of the substance divided by the product of the concentration of the substance and the absorption path length, and according to the SI should be expressed in m^2 per mole. The terms formerly used for molar absorptivity include molar absorbancy index and molar extinction coefficient.

Absorption spectrum — The relationship of absorbance and wavelength or any functions of these, frequently represented in a graphic form.

The use of absorption spectrophotometry in the visible and ultraviolet regions for assay procedures is based on the fact that the absorptivity of a substance is usually a constant independent of the intensity of the incident radiation, the internal cell length, and the concentration, with the result that concentration may be determined photometrically.

Deviations from the above may be caused by either physical, chemical, or instrumental variables. Deviations due to instrumental error might be caused by slit-width effects, stray light, or by polychromatic radiation. Apparent failure may also result from a concentration change in solute molecules because of association between solute molecules or between solute and solvent molecules, or dissociation or ionization.

Apparatus

In essence all types of spectrophotometer are designed to permit substantially monochromatic radiant energy to be passed through the test substance in a suitable form and to allow measurement of the fraction of that energy that is transmitted. The spectrophotometer comprises an energy source, a dispersing device with slits for selecting the wavelength band, a cell or holder for the test substance, a detector of radiant energy, associated amplifiers, and measuring and recording devices. Some instruments are manually operated, while others are equipped for automatic operation. Instruments are available for use in the visible region of the spectrum, usually 380 nm to about 700 nm, and in the visible and ultraviolet regions of the spectrum, usually 190 nm to about 700 nm.

Both double-beam and single-beam instruments are commercially available and either is suitable. Depending on the type of apparatus used, the results may be displayed on a scale, on a digital counter, or by a recorder or printer.

The apparatus should be maintained in proper working condition. The housing of the optical system should minimize any possibility of errors due to stray light; this is particularly relevant in the short-wave region of the spectrum.

Cells usually used in the spectral range discussed are 1-cm absorption cells with glass or silica windows. Other path lengths may also be used. The cells used for the test solution and the blank should be matched, and must have the same spectral transmittance when containing only the solvent. If this is not the case, an appropriate correction must be applied.

Spectrophotometer calibration

Spectrophotometers should be regularly checked for accuracy of calibrations. Where a continuous source of radiant energy is used, both the wavelength and photometric scales should be calibrated; where a spectral line source is used, only the photometric scale need be checked.

A number of sources of radiant energy have spectral lines of suitable intensity, adequately spaced throughout the spectral range selected. The exact values for the position of characteristic lines in quartz-mercury arc are 253.7, 302.25, 313.16, 334.15, 365.48, 404.66 and 435.83 nm. The wavelength scale may also be calibrated by means of suitable glass filters that have useful absorption bands through the visible and ultraviolet regions. Standard glass containing didymium (a mixture of praseodymium and neodymium) has been widely used. Glass containing holmium is considered superior. The exact values for the position of characteristic maxima in holmium glass filters are 241.5 ± 1, 287.5 ± 1,

360.9 $\pm$ 1 and 536.2 $\pm$ 3 nm. Holmium glass filters are obtainable from some national institutions and from commercial sources. The performance of an uncertified filter should be checked against one that has been properly certified. The wavelength scale may also be calibrated using holmium perchlorate TS. The exact values for the position of characteristic maxima of this solution are as follows: 241.15 nm, 278.2 nm, 361.5 nm and 536.3 nm. It should be noted that the position of characteristic maxima of holmium perchlorate solutions and holmium glass filters may differ slightly.

For the calibration of the photometric scale the tolerance generally permitted is $\pm$ 1 % of the absorptivity. For checking this scale potassium dichromate TS may be used. The exact values of absorbance and specific extinction for a solution of potassium dichromate containing exactly 60.06 mg in 1000 ml of sulfuric acid (0.005 mol/l) VS at an absorption path length of 1.000 cm and the permitted tolerances for A are given below:

Wavelength	235 nm (minimum)	257 nm (maximum)	313 nm (minimum)	350 nm (maximum)
A	0.748	0.865	0.292	0.640
Permitted tolerance	0.740-0.756	0.856-0.874	0.289-0.295	0.634-0.646
$E^{1\ \%}_{1\ cm}$	124.54	144.02	48.62	106.56

A number of standard inorganic glass filters of known transmittance produced for checking the photometric scale are also available from some national institutions and from commercial sources but may require periodic calibration.

Operation of spectrophotometers

Detailed instructions for operating spectrophotometers are supplied by the manufacturers. To achieve significant and valid results, the operator of a spectrophotometer should be aware of its limitations and of potential sources of error and variation. The instruction manual should be followed closely on such matters as care, cleaning, and calibration of the instrument, and instructions for operation. Where double-beam recording instruments are used the cell containing solvent only is placed in the reference beam.

The cleanliness of absorption cells should receive particular attention. Usually, after treatment with an appropriate cleansing medium, the cells should be rinsed with distilled water and then with a volatile organic solvent to promote drying. Test solutions should not be left in the cells longer than necessary for carrying out the measurement. When handling the cells, special care should be taken never to touch the external surfaces through which the light beam passes. When the solvent and the test solution are transferred to the cells, care is to be taken that the liquids do not contaminate the outer surfaces.

Solvents for use in the ultraviolet region

Many solvents are suitable for tests and assays using spectrophotometry in the ultraviolet region. Water, alcohols, chloroform, lower hydrocarbons, ethers, and dilute solutions of ammonium hydroxide, sodium hydroxide, sulfuric acid and hydrochloric acid can be used for this purpose. The solvents differ as to the lower wavelength at which the decrease in transparency prevents their use. Precautions should be taken to use solvents free from contaminants absorbing in the relevant spectral region. Specially purified solvents for spectrophotometric determinations are available commercially from several sources but need only be used when the spectral characteristics of the usual analytical grade of solvent are inadequate for a particular purpose.

The absorbance of the solvent cell and its contents should not exceed 0.4 per cm of path length when measured with reference to air at the same wavelength. The solvent in the solvent cell should be of the same batch as that used to prepare the solution and must be free from fluorescence at the wavelength of measurement. Ethanol ($\sim$750 g/l), dehydrated ethanol, methanol, and cyclohexane used as solvents should have an absorbance, measured in a 1-cm cell at 240 nm with reference to water, not exceeding 0.10.

Identification tests in the ultraviolet region

The monographs describing qualitative tests involving spectrophotometry in the ultraviolet region specify the concentration of the solution and the path length. In such tests it is more convenient to use a recording instrument. If the conditions stated are not appropriate for a particular instrument, the thickness of the solution should be varied and not the concentration.

Some identification tests involving spectrophotometry require the use of reference substances, generally an International Chemical Reference Substance. The reference substance is then to be prepared and simultaneously measured under conditions identical for all practical purposes to those used for the test substance. Unless otherwise specified in the monograph, in making up the solution of the reference substance, a solution of about the desired concentration (i.e. within 10 % of the value) should be prepared. Identical conditions for the measurement include the following: wavelength setting, slit-width adjustment, cell placement, and correction and transmittance levels.

A useful approach for identification tests in the ultraviolet region is to quote the ratio of absorbance values at two maxima. This procedure minimizes the influence of instrumental variations on the test and obviates the need for a reference substance.

Quantitative determinations in the ultraviolet region

Spectrophotometric assays usually call for a comparison of the absorbance produced by the solution of the test substance, prepared as specified in the monograph, with the absorbance of a solution of a reference substance. In such cases the spectrophotometric measurements are made first with the solution prepared from the reference substance and secondly with the solution prepared from the substance to be examined. The second measurement is carried out as quickly as possible after the first, using the same experimental conditions.

Spectrophotometric assays are usually carried out at a peak of spectral absorption for the compound concerned. The monographs give the commonly accepted wavelength for peak spectral absorption of the substance in question. It is known that different spectrophotometers may show minor variations in the apparent wavelength of this peak. Good practice demands that use be made of the peak wavelength actually found in the individual instrument, rather than the specific wavelength given in the monograph, provided the two do not differ by more than $\pm$ 0.5 nm in the 240–280 nm range, by more than $\pm$ 1 nm in the 280–320 nm range, and by more than $\pm$ 2 nm above 320 nm. If the difference is greater, recalibration of the instrument may be indicated.

The solution of the reference substance, generally an International Chemical Reference Substance, is to be prepared and measured in the same manner as described for "Identification tests in the ultraviolet region". The calculations should be made on the basis of the exact amount weighed and, if the reference substance used has not previously been dried, on the dried or anhydrous basis. Specific instructions in individual monographs indicate the manner in which a reference substance is to be dried or treated prior to use. These instructions are to be followed unless otherwise specified in the individual test or assay, or in the labelling.

To ensure that the conditions used are appropriate the monograph may also specify the value of absorbance of a 1-cm layer of the reference substance. In this case the determination carried out against the reference substance is considered valid when the observed value of absorbance is within the range of values specified in the monograph.

For quantitative work, a manually scanning instrument is frequently used. When a recording instrument is used for that purpose special attention should be paid to proper calibration of the absorbance scale at the wavelength used.

Quantitative determinations are usually carried out at wavelengths above 235 nm. If the measurements are to be made at a wavelength in the 190–210 nm range, special precautions should be observed, for example, purging the cell compartment with nitrogen, use of solvents of special spectrophotometric quality, and using cells that are transparent in this region.

When measuring the absorbance at an absorption maximum the spectral slit-width must be small compared with the half width of the absorption band, otherwise an erroneously low absorbance will be measured. Particular care is needed for certain substances and the instrumental slit-width used should always be such that further reduction does not result in an increased absorbance reading. Problems may be encountered, owing to diffraction of the light beam, at slit-widths below 0.01 mm.

When the assays are carried out with routine frequency it is permissible to omit the use of a reference substance and use instead a suitable standard curve prepared with the respective International Chemical Reference Substance. This may be done when, for the substance tested, the absorbance is proportional to the concentration within the range of about 75–125 % of the final concentration used in the assay. Under these circumstances, the absorbance found in the assay may be interpolated on the standard curve, and the assay result calculated therefrom. Such standard curves should be confirmed frequently, and always when a new apparatus or new lots of reagents are put into use. In the event of uncertainty or dispute, direct comparison with an International Chemical Reference Substance must be made.

Quantitative determinations in the visible region

Spectrophotometric assays in the visible region, as in the ultraviolet region, usually call for simultaneous comparison of the absorbance produced by the assay preparation with that produced by a standard preparation containing approximately an equal quantity of a reference substance.

For spectrophotometric assays in the visible region the recommendations given under "Quantitative determinations in the ultraviolet region", including those concerning the use of standard curves, should be followed with suitable modifications, where necessary. In this region, observed wavelengths should not differ by more than 5 nm from that specified in the monograph.

SPECTROPHOTOMETRY IN THE INFRARED REGION

The infrared region of the electromagnetic spectrum used in pharmaceutical analysis covers the range 4000–250 cm^{-1} (2.5–40 μm).[1]

Spectrophotometric measurements in the infrared region are used mainly as an identification test. The infrared spectrum is unique for any given chemical compound with the exception of optical isomers, which have identical spectra in solution. Polymorphism and other factors, such as variations in crystal size and orientation, the grinding procedure, and the possible formation of hydrates may, however, be responsible for a difference in the infrared spectrum of a given compound in the solid state. The infrared spectrum is usually not greatly affected by the presence of small quantities of impurities (up to several percent) in the tested substance. For identification purposes the spectrum may be compared with that of a reference substance, concomitantly prepared or with a standard reference spectrum.

The terms *absorption spectrum, absorbance, transmittance, absorptivity,* and *specific extinction* are described in "Spectrophotometry in the visible and ultraviolet regions" (see page 33).

Apparatus

Spectrophotometers for the infrared region are basically similar to those used for the visible and ultraviolet regions of the spectrum, but may differ as to the energy sources, optical materials, and detection devices. Furthermore, in some instruments the monochromator may be located between the test substance and the detector.

Spectrophotometers suitable for use for identification tests should operate in the range 4000–670 cm^{-1} (2.5–15 μm). They should be checked frequently to ensure that they meet the standards of performance laid down by the manufacturer of the instrument, including the reliability of the wavelength scales, which should be checked by use of a polystyrene film.

For the use of the attenuated total reflectance technique, the instrument should be equipped with a suitable attachment, which may be a single-reflection or a multi-reflection one. The attachment consists of a reflecting element and a suitable mounting permitting its alignment in the spectrophotometer for maximum transmission.

---

[1] The values given in brackets are wavelengths; the preceding values are wavenumbers, which are the reciprocals of the wavelengths.

Use of solvents

The solvent used in infrared spectrophotometry must not affect the material, usually sodium chloride, of which the cell is made.

No solvent in appreciable thickness is completely transparent throughout the infrared spectrum. Carbon tetrachloride R is practically transparent (up to 1 mm in thickness) from 4000 to 1700 cm^{-1} (2.5 to 6 μm). Chloroform R, dichloromethane R, and dibromomethane R are other useful solvents. Carbon disulfide IR (up to 1 mm in thickness) is suitable as a solvent to 250 cm^{-1} (40 μm), except in the 2400–2000 cm^{-1} (4.2–5.0 μm) and the 1800–1300 cm^{-1} (5.5–7.5 μm) regions, where it has strong absorption. Its weak absorption in the 875–845 cm^{-1} (11.4–11.8 μm) region should also be noted. Other solvents have relatively narrow regions of transparency.

Preparation of the substance to be tested

To determine the infrared absorption spectrum of a substance, the latter has to be suitably prepared. Liquid substances may be tested directly or in a suitable solution. For solid substances, the usual methods of preparation include dispersing the finely ground solid specimen in mineral oil, or incorporating it in a transparent disc or pellet obtained by mixing it intimately with previously dried potassium halide and pressing the mixture in a die, or preparing a solution in a suitable solvent. Preparation of the substance for the attenuated total reflectance technique is described separately.

The following procedures may be used for the preparation of the substance:

Method 1. Use a capillary film of the liquid held between two sodium chloride plates or a filled cell of suitable thickness.

Method 2. Triturate a small quantity of the substance with the minimum amount of a suitable mineral oil or other suitable liquid to give a smooth, creamy paste; 2–5 mg of the substance being tested is often sufficient to prepare a satisfactory mull, which should be semi-transparent to light. Compress a portion of the mull between two flat sodium chloride or other suitable plates.

Method 3. Triturate the solid substance with dry, finely powdered potassium halide (potassium bromide IR, potassium chloride IR); the proportion of substance to the halide should be about 1 to 200 —, for example, 1.5 mg in 300 mg of the halide — in the case of prism instruments, and about 1 to 300 — for example, 1.0 mg in 300 mg of the halide — in the case of grating instruments. The amount taken should be such that the weight of substance per area of the disc is about 5–15 μg per mm^2, varying with the molecular weight and to some degree with the type of apparatus used. Insert a portion of the mixture in a special die and subject it under vacuum to a high pressure. Commercial dies are available and the manufacturer's instructions should be followed. Mount the resultant disc in a suitable holder. Several factors, for example, inadequate or excessive grinding, moisture or other impurities in the halide carrier, may give rise to unsatisfactory discs. Unless its preparation presents particular difficulties, a disc should be rejected if visual inspection shows lack of uniformity or if the transmission at about 2000 cm^{-1} (5 μm) in the absence of a specific absorption band is less than 75 % without compensation.

Method 4. Prepare a solution of the liquid or solid substance in a suitable solvent and choose a concentration and cell thickness to give a satisfactory spectrum over a sufficiently wide wavelength range.

Identification by reference substance

Prepare the substance under examination and the reference substance by the same method, and record the spectrum of each from about 4000 to 670 cm^{-1} (2.5 μm to 15 μm) on an infrared spectrophotometer. The concentration of the substance should be such that the strongest peak attributable to the substance reaches to between 5 % and 25 % transmittance.

If the positions and relative intensities of the absorbance maxima in the spectrum of the substance under examination are not concordant with those of the spectrum of the reference substance in the case of the curves obtained by methods 2 or 3, this may be due to differences in crystalline form. When such difficulties are suspected, the substance should, where possible, be examined in solution. If examination in solution is not practicable, attempts should be made to obtain, by recrystallization, the reference substance and the substance under examination in the same crystalline form.

If the spectrum of mineral oil used in method 2 interferes with regions of interest, an additional dispersion of the substance in a medium such as a suitable fluorinated hydrocarbon oil or hexachlorobutadiene may be prepared and the spectrum recorded in the regions where the mineral oil shows strong absorption.

Identification by reference spectrum

Prepare the substance being examined exactly as described in the note accompanying the International Reference Spectrum and record the spectrum from about 4000 to 670 cm^{-1} (2.5 to 15 μm) using an instrument that is being checked frequently to ensure that it meets the standards of performance laid down by the manufacturer. To allow for a possible difference in wavelength calibration between the instrument on which the International Reference Spectrum was obtained and that on which the spectrum of the substance is to be recorded, reference absorbance maxima of a polystyrene spectrum are superimposed on the International Reference Spectrum at about 2851 cm^{-1} (3.51 μm), 1601 cm^{-1} (6.25 μm) and 1028 cm^{-1} (9.73 μm). Similar reference maxima should be superimposed on the spectrum of the substance. Taking these polystyrene maxima into account, the identification is considered to be positive if the principal absorbance maxima in the spectrum of the substance being tested are concordant with the corresponding maxima in the relevant International Reference Spectrum. When comparing the two spectra, care should be taken to allow for the possibility of differences in resolving power between the instrument on which the International Reference Spectrum was prepared and the instrument being used to examine the substance. An International Reference Spectrum of polystyrene that was recorded on the same instrument as the collection of International Reference Spectra should be used for assessing these differences. It should be noted that the greatest variation due to differences in resolving power is likely to occur in the region between 4000 and 2000 cm^{-1} (2.5 and 5 μm).

Attenuated total reflectance technique

To determine the infrared absorption spectrum of a substance by the attenuated total reflectance technique the solid substance has usually to be finely pulverized. The powder may then be either packed directly against the prism of the attachment or adhesive tape may be used to facilitate the contact. The powdered substance is spread on the adhesive side of an adhesive tape to form an almost translucent layer and the tape is pressed on the reflecting element, on the side with powder in contact. Next, either the backing plate is attached or moderate pressure is applied in a suitable clamp for 1–2 minutes. Finally, the reflecting element is placed in the holder. The tape used in the procedure should preferably contain a natural rubber adhesive. In the case of some plastic materials it may be placed directly on the reflecting element.

Proper alignment of the attachment in the apparatus should be carefully controlled.

ATOMIC ABSORPTION SPECTROPHOTOMETRY

Flame atomic absorption spectrophotometry, or flame absorption spectrophotometry, is a procedure during which atoms, ions, or ion complexes of an element, upon being atomized to the ground state in a flame, absorb light at the characteristic wavelength for that element.

If the absorption process takes place in the flame under reproducible conditions, the absorbance (the reciprocal logarithm of the transmittance) is proportional to the number of absorbing atoms. On this basis, calibration curves may be constructed to permit evaluation of unknown absorption values in terms of concentration of the element in solution.

It may be noted that besides flame atomic absorption spectrophotometry, flameless techniques of atomic absorption spectrophotometry have also been evolved.

Apparatus

A flame atomic absorption spectrophotometer consists of an emission source that provides the characteristic spectral line of the element to be determined, a nebulizer-burner system for introducing the sample solution into a flame, and a detector system.

The emission source is usually a hollow-cathode discharge lamp, the cathode of which is designed to emit the desired radiation when excited. Since the radiation to be absorbed by the element in the test solution is usually of the same wavelength as that of its emission line, the element in the hollow-cathode lamp will be the same as the element to be determined. In general, a different lamp is used for each element; however, some element combinations are compatible with single lamps now available commercially.

The nebulizer-burner system introduces the test solution into a flame, which is usually provided by air-acetylene or air-hydrogen. The flame, in effect, is a heated sample chamber.

The detector system used to read the signal from the chamber is composed of an optical dispersing device, such as a monochromator or a filter for isolating a resonance line of the element, and a radiation detector, such as a photomultiplier and display system to indicate the absorbance.

Interfering radiation produced by the flame during combustion may be negated by the use of a chopped source lamp signal of a definite frequency. The detector should then be tuned to the alternating current frequency so that the direct current signal arising from the flame will be ignored. Such a detecting system, therefore, reads only the change in signal from the hollow-cathode source, which is directly proportional to the number of atoms to be determined in the substance.

Use of solvents

An ideal solvent is one that interferes to a minimal extent in the absorption or emission processes and one that produces neutral atoms in the flame. If there is a significant difference between the surface tension or viscosity of the substance and those of the reference solution, the solutions will be aspirated or atomized at different rates, causing significant differences in the signals generated. The acid concentration of the solutions also affects the absorption process. Therefore, the solvent used in preparing the test solution and that used for the reference solution should be either the same or as much alike as possible in these respects, and should yield solutions that are easily aspirated via the tube of the burner-aspirator. Where solids are present in solutions they may give rise to interferences and for that reason the solid content of the solutions should be below 2 % wherever possible.

RECOMMENDED PROCEDURE

Prepare not fewer than 3 reference solutions of the element to be determined covering the concentration range recommended by the manufacturers for the element and instrument used. Any reagent used in preparing the solution of the substance being examined should be added to the reference solutions in the same concentration.

For measurements on instruments calibrated for transmission, spray water into the flame and adjust the reading to full scale; no further adjustments are necessary for this type of instrument. For instruments calibrated for absorption, refer to the manufacturer's instructions. Spray each reference solution into the flame 3 times, recording the steady reading obtained and washing the apparatus through with water after each spraying. Prepare a calibration curve by plotting the mean of each group of 3 readings against the concentration.

Prepare a solution of the substance being examined as specified in the monograph but adjust the concentration of the element to be determined, if necessary, so that it falls within the concentration range recommended for the instrument used. Spray the solution into the flame 3 times, record the readings and wash the apparatus through with water after each spraying. Use the mean of the readings to determine the concentration of the element from the calibration curve.

FLUORESCENCE SPECTROPHOTOMETRY

Fluorescence spectrophotometry is the measurement of the fluorescence, i.e., photoluminescence, emitted by a substance while it is being exposed to ultraviolet, visible, or other electromagnetic radiation. In general, the light emitted by fluorescent solutions is of maximum intensity at a wavelength longer than that of the absorption band causing excitation, usually by some 20 or 30 nm.

The intensity of the light emitted by a fluorescent solution is, in certain circumstances, a simple function of the concentration of the solute and can, therefore, be used for analysis. It is difficult, however, to measure absolute fluorescence intensity, and measurements are usually made by reference to dilutions of a properly selected reference substance. The general scheme in fluorescence spectroscopy is therefore to excite with radiation at the wavelength of maximum absorption, and to measure or compare the intensity of the fluorescent light with that of a reference solution. The fluorescent light should be carefully freed from scattered incident light.

Terms

Fluorescence intensity is an empirical expression of fluorescence activity, commonly given in terms of arbitrary units proportional to detector response.

The *fluorescence emission spectrum* is the relationship between the intensity of the emitted radiation and the wavelength and is frequently represented in a graphic form.

The *fluorescence excitation spectrum* is the relationship between the maximum intensity of radiation emitted by an activated substance and the wavelength of the incident radiation and is frequently represented in a graphic form.

Apparatus

Measurement of fluorescence intensity can be made with a simple filter fluorimeter (sometimes the term fluorometer is used). Such an instrument consists of a radiation source, a primary filter, a sample chamber, a secondary filter, and a fluorescence detection system. In most such fluorimeters, the detector is placed on an axis at 90° from that of the incident beam. This right-angle geometry permits the incident radiation to pass through the test solution without contaminating the output signal received by the fluorescence detector. However, the detector unavoidably receives some of the incident radiation as a result of the inherent scattering properties of the solutions themselves, or if dust or other solids are present. Filters are used to eliminate this residual scatter. The primary filter selects short wavelength radiation capable of causing excitation of the test substance, while the secondary filter is normally a sharp cut-off filter that allows the longer wavelength fluorescence to be transmitted but blocks the scattered excited radiation.

Most fluorimeters use photomultiplier tubes as detectors; many types are available, each having special characteristics with respect to spectral region of maximum sensitivity, gain, and electrical noise. After amplification of the photocurrent its value is read visually on a measuring device or recorded.

A fluorescence spectrophotometer differs from a filter fluorimeter in that filters are replaced by monochromators, of either the prism or the grating type. For analytical purposes, the fluorescence spectrophotometer is superior to the filter fluorimeter in wavelength selectivity, flexibility, and convenience.

Many radiation sources are used in fluorimeters and fluorescence spectrophotometers. Mercury lamps are relatively stable and emit energy mainly at discrete wavelengths. Tungsten lamps provide an energy continuum in the visible region. The high pressure xenon arc lamp is often used in fluorescence spectrophotometers because it has an energy continuum extending from the ultraviolet into the infrared.

In fluorescence spectrophotometers the monochromators are equipped with slits. A narrow slit provides high resolution and spectral purity, while a large slit sacrifices these for high intensity. Choice of slit-width is determined by the wavelength separation between incident and emitted radiation, as well as by the degree of sensitivity needed.

The cells used in fluorescence measurements may be rectangular cells similar to those used in absorption spectrophotometers, except that they are polished on all 4 vertical sides and on the bottom, or cells in the shape of round tubes with flat polished bottoms may be used. A convenient size is 2–3 ml, but some instruments can be fitted with small cells holding 0.1–0.3 ml, or with a capillary holder requiring even less solution.

Standardization

Fluorimeters and fluorescence spectrophotometers should be standardized daily with a stable fluorophore to assure proper reproducibility of response. The changes are due to instrumental variables such as differences in lamp intensity and photomultiplier sensitivity. The fluorophore may be a pure specimen of the fluorescent substance under test or another readily purified fluorescent substance with absorption and fluorescence bands similar to those of the test substance. Quinine in dilute sulfuric acid is often a convenient fluorophore for blue fluorescence, sodium fluorescein for green fluorescence, and rhodamine for red fluorescence.

Calibration of the wavelength scale

The wavelength scale of the fluorescence spectrophotometer should be periodically calibrated.

Preparation of solution

The solvent used for the measurement should be properly selected. The solvent itself, its purity and its pH may markedly affect the intensity and spectral distribution of fluorescence.

Test solutions prepared for fluorescence spectrophotometry are usually 10 times to 100 times less concentrated than those used in absorption spectrophotometry. In analytical applications, it is necessary that the fluorescence intensity be linearly related to the concentration in the range used for measurements; but if a solution is too concentrated, a significant part of the incident light is absorbed by the substance near the cell surface, thus resulting in a reduction of the light reaching the centre. That is, the substance itself acts as an "inner filter". Fortunately, fluorescence spectrophotometry is inherently a very sensitive technique, and concentrations of 10^{-5}–10^{-7} mol/l are frequently used.

Owing to the usually very narrow range within which the fluorescence is proportional to the concentration of the fluorescent substance, the ratio $(c—d)/(a—b)$, where a is the fluorescence intensity read for the reference substance, b the reading for the corresponding blank, c the fluorescence intensity read for the test substance, and d the reading for the corresponding blank, should be not less than 0.40 and not more than 2.50. It is then necessary to make a working curve of fluorescence intensity corrected for a solvent blank versus concentration.

Measurement technique

Fluorescence measurements are sensitive to the presence of solid particles in the test solution. Such impurities may reduce the intensity of the exciting beam or give misleadingly high readings because of multiple reflections in the cell. It is, therefore, wise to eliminate solid particles by centrifugation; filtration may also be used, but some filter-papers may contain fluorescent impurities.

Oxygen dissolved in the solvent has a strong quenching effect. The intensity of fluorescence is therefore increased by use of a degassing procedure, such as bubbling nitrogen or another inert gas through the test solution.

Temperature regulation is often important in fluorescence spectrophotometry. For some substances, fluorescence efficiency may be reduced by as much as 1–2 % per degree of temperature rise. In such cases, if maximum precision is desired, temperature-controlled sample cells are essential. For routine analysis, it may be sufficient to make measurements rapidly enough so that the test solution does not heat up appreciably from exposure to the intense light source.

Many fluorescent compounds are light-sensitive. Exposed in a fluorescence spectrophotometer, they may be photodegraded into more or less fluorescent products. Such effects may be detected by observing the detector response in relation to time, and may be reduced by attenuating the light source with filters or screens.

TURBIDIMETRY AND NEPHELOMETRY

Turbidimetry is the measurement of the degree of attenuation of a radiant beam incident on particles suspended in a medium, the measurement being made in the directly transmitted beam. It may be measured with a standard photoelectric filter photometer or spectrophotometer with illumination at an appropriate wavelength.

Nephelometry is the measurement of the light scattered by suspended particles, the measurement usually being made perpendicularly to the incident beam.

Turbidimetry or nephelometry may be useful for the measurement of precipitates formed by the interaction of very dilute solutions of reagents, or other particulate matter, such as suspensions of bacterial cells. In order that consistent results may be achieved, all variables must be carefully controlled. Problems due to birefringence may be encountered, particularly with bacterial cells. Where proper control is possible, extremely dilute suspensions may be measured.

Terms

Transmittance (T) — The ratio of the radiant flux transmitted by the test substance to that of the incident radiant flux. Terms formerly used include transmittancy and transmission.

Turbidance (S) — A measure of the light-scattering effect of suspended particles.

Turbidity (τ) — In light-scattering measurements, the turbidity is the measure of the decrease in incident beam intensity per unit length of a given suspension.

Apparatus

Turbidity may be measured with a standard photoelectric filter photometer or spectrophotometer, preferably with illumination in the red-orange region of the spectrum (for example, by using a blue filter).

Nephelometric measurements require an instrument with a photocell placed so as to receive scattered rather than transmitted light; as this geometry applies also to fluorimeters in general, the latter can be used as nephelometers by proper selection of filters.

Instrumental measurement

For instrumental measurement it is advisable to ensure that settling of the particles being measured will be negligible. This is usually accomplished by including a protective colloid in the liquid suspending medium. It is important that results be interpreted by comparison of readings with those representing known concentrations of suspended matter, produced under exactly the same conditions.

Visual comparison

Carry out turbidity comparison in tubes that are matched as closely as possible in internal diameter and in all other respects. Flat-bottomed comparison tubes of transparent glass of about 70 ml capacity and about 23 mm internal diameter are suitable. For turbidity comparison the tubes should be viewed horizontally, against a dark background, with the aid of a light source directed from the sides of the tubes.

COLOUR OF LIQUIDS

The test for colour of liquids is carried out by comparing the test solution prepared as specified in the monograph with a standard colour solution indicated in the monograph. The composition of the standard colour solution is selected depending on the hue and intensity of the colour of the test solution corresponding to the limits permitted in the specifications.

RECOMMENDED PROCEDURE

Unless otherwise specified in the monograph, carry out the comparison in flat-bottomed tubes of transparent glass that are matched as closely as possible in internal diameter and in all other respects (tubes of about 16 mm internal diameter are suitable). Use 10 ml of the test solution and 10 ml of the standard colour solution; the depth of liquid should be about 50 mm. The colour of the test solution is not more intense than the standard colour when viewed down the vertical axis of the tubes in diffused light against a white background.

Stock Colour Standard Solutions

Yellow stock standard TS

To 9.5 ml of cobalt colour TS, add 1.9 ml of copper colour TS, 10.7 ml of dichromate colour TS, 4.0 ml of iron colour TS, dilute to 100.0 ml with sulfuric acid (~10 g/l) TS, and mix.

Red stock standard TS

To 40.5 ml of cobalt colour TS, add 6.1 ml of copper colour TS, 6.3 ml of dichromate colour TS, 12.0 ml of iron colour TS, dilute to 100.0 ml with sulfuric acid (~10 g/l) TS, and mix.

Green stock standard TS

To 3.5 ml of cobalt colour TS, add 20.1 ml of copper colour TS, 10.4 ml of dichromate colour TS, 4.0 ml of iron colour TS, dilute to 100.0 ml with sulfuric acid (~10 g/l) TS, and mix.

Brown stock standard TS

To 35.0 ml of cobalt colour TS, add 17.0 ml of copper colour TS, 8.0 ml of dichromate colour TS, dilute to 100.0 ml with iron colour TS, and mix.

Standard Colour Solutions

The standard colour solution is prepared by suitably diluting the stock standard solutions (yellow, red, green, and brown stock standard TS) with sulfuric acid (~10 g/l) TS. The designation of the standard colour solution is composed of two letters indicating the stock standard solution (Yw for yellow, Rd for red, Gn for green, and Bn for brown) and of a number describing the dilution, as given below :

Dilution number for standard colour solutions	Stock standard solution (ml)	Sulfuric acid (~10 g/l) TS (ml)
0	0.78	99.22
1	1.56	98.44
2	3.12	96.88
3	6.25	93.75
4	12.50	87.50
5	25.00	75.00
6	50.00	50.00
7	100.00	—

Standard colour solution numbers 4–7 may be stored in sealed glass containers, protected from sunlight but the more dilute standard colour solutions should be prepared as required.

RADIOPHARMACEUTICALS

The handling and testing of radiopharmaceuticals (radioactive pharmaceuticals) require specialized techniques in order that correct results may be obtained and hazards to personnel minimized. All operations should be carried out or supervised by personnel who have received expert training in handling radioactive materials.

Definitions

Nuclide

A species of atom characterized by its mass number, atomic number, and nuclear energy state, provided that the mean life in that state is long enough to be observable.

Radioactivity

The property of certain nuclides of emitting radiation by the spontaneous transformation of their nuclei into those of other nuclides.

EXPLANATORY NOTE. The term "desintegration" is widely used as an alternative to the term "transformation". Transformation is preferred as it includes, without semantic difficulties, those processes in which no particles are emitted from the nucleus.

Radionuclide

A nuclide that is radioactive.

Units of radioactivity

The activity of a quantity of radioactive material is expressed in terms of the number of nuclear transformations taking place in unit time. The SI unit of activity is the becquerel (Bq), a special name for the reciprocal second (s^{-1}). The expression of activity in terms of the becquerel therefore indicates the number of disintegrations per second. One curie (Ci) equals 3.7×10^{10} Bq.

The conversion factors between becquerel and curie and its submultiples are given in "Units of measurement" (see page 14).

Half-life period

The time in which the radioactivity decreases to one-half its original value.

EXPLANATORY NOTE. The rate of radioactive decay is constant and characteristic for each individual radionuclide. The exponential decay curve is described mathematically by the equation

$$N = N_0 e^{-\lambda t}$$

where N is the number of atoms at elapsed time t, N_0 is the number of atoms when $t = 0$, and λ is the disintegration constant characteristic of each individual radionuclide. The half-life period is related to the disintegration constant by the equation

$$T_{\frac{1}{2}} = \frac{0.693}{\lambda}$$

Radioactive decay corrections are calculated from the exponential equation, or from decay tables, or are obtained from a decay curve plotted for the particular radionuclide involved (see Fig. 1).

FIG. 1. MASTER DECAY CHART

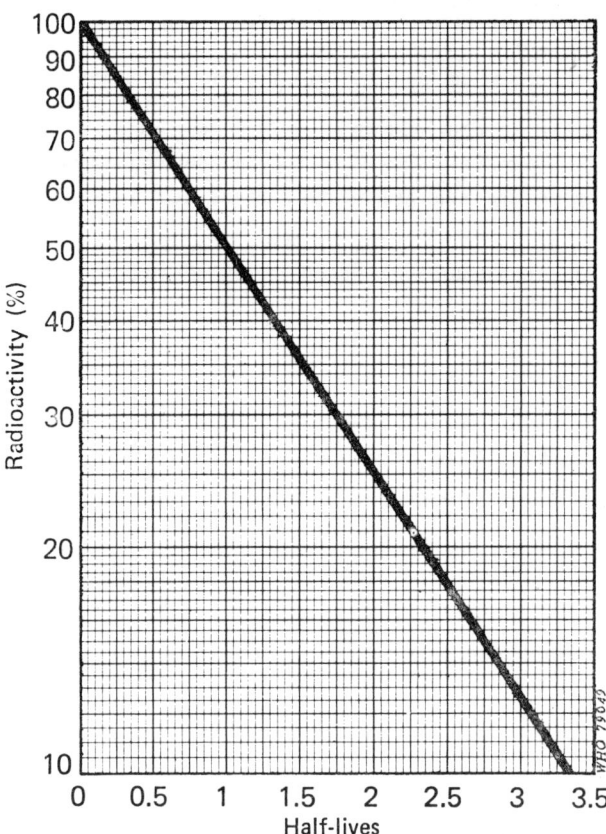

Radioactive concentration

The radioactive concentration of a solution refers to the radioactivity in a unit volume of the solution. As with all statements involving radioactivity, it is necessary to include a reference date of standardization. For radionuclides with a half-life period of less than 30 days, the time of standardization should be expressed to the nearest hour. For radionuclides with a half-life period of less than one day, a more precise statement of the reference time is required.

Specific radioactivity (or specific activity)

The specific activity of a preparation of a radioactive material is the radioactivity per unit mass of the element or of the compound concerned.

EXPLANATORY NOTE. It is usual to specify the radionuclide concerned and also it is necessary to express the time thus: "1 mCi of iodine-131 per mg of o-iodohippuric acid at 12.00 hours UT on 1 January 1979", or "40 MBq of selenium-75 per mg of selenomethionine on 1 January 1979".

Specific radioactivity is often not determined directly but is calculated from a knowledge of the radioactive concentration of the solution and of the chemical concentration of the radioactive compound. Thus, if a solution contains x mCi of ^{131}I per ml, and if the ^{131}I is entirely in the chemical form of sodium o-iodohippurate of which the concentration is y mg per ml, then at that time the specific activity is:

$$x/y \text{ mCi of iodine-131 per mg of } o\text{-iodohippuric acid.}$$

Where necessary, the radiochemical purity of the preparation (see below) must be taken into account.

The term employed in radiochemical work is "specific activity". As the word, "activity" has other connotations in a pharmacopoeia, the term should, where necessary, be modified to "specific radioactivity" to avoid ambiguity.

Radionuclidic purity

The radionuclidic purity of a preparation is that percentage of the total radioactivity that is present in the form of the stated radionuclide.

EXPLANATORY NOTE. Some radionuclides decay into nuclides that are themselves radioactive: these are referred to as mother (or parent) and daughter radionuclides respectively. Such daughter radionuclides are often excluded when calculating the radionuclidic purity; for example, iodine-131 will always contain its daughter xenon-131m, but this would not be considered an impurity because its presence is unavoidable.

In employing the definition, the radioactivity must be measured in appropriate units: that is, in the number of nuclear transformations that occur in unit time (in terms of curies or becquerels). If, for example, a preparation stated to be iodine-125 is known to contain 99 mCi of iodine-125 and 1 mCi of iodine-126, and no other radionuclide, then the preparation is said to be of 99 % radionuclidic purity. It will be noted that the relative amounts of iodine-125 and iodine-126, and hence the radionuclidic purity, will change with time. An expression of radionuclidic purity must therefore contain a statement of the time, such as: "Not more than 1 % of the total radioactivity is due to iodine-126 at the reference date stated on the label". In the case of radionuclides with a half-life period of less than 30 days the reference hour should also be included.

It is clear that, in order to give a statement of the radionuclidic purity of a preparation, the activities (and hence the identities) of every radionuclide present must be known. There are no simple and certain means of identifying and measuring all the radionuclidic impurities that might be present in a preparation. An expression of radionuclidic purity must either depend upon the judgement of the person concerned, or it must be qualified by reference to the method employed, for example : "No radionuclidic impurities were detected by gamma scintillation spectrometry using a sodium iodide detector."

Radiochemical purity

The radiochemical purity of a preparation is that percentage of the stated radionuclide that is present in the stated chemical form. As radiochemical purity may change with time, mainly because of radiation decomposition, the time at which the radiochemical purity limit is applicable must be specified.

EXPLANATORY NOTE. If, for example, a preparation of cyanocobalamin (^{57}Co) is stated to be 99 % radiochemically pure, then 99 % of the cobalt-57 is present in the form of cyanocobalamin. Radiochemical impurities might include such substances as cobaltous (^{57}Co) ion or hydroxycobalamin (^{57}Co).

The possible presence of radionuclidic impurities is not taken into account in the definition. If the radionuclidic impurity is not isotopic with the stated radionuclide, then it cannot possibly be in the identical chemical form. If the radionuclidic impurity is isotopic with the stated radionuclide, it could be, and indeed is likely to be, in the same chemical form.

Radiochemical impurities may arise during the preparation of the material or during storage, because of ordinary chemical decomposition or, what is often more important, because of radiation decomposition (that is, because of the physical and chemical effects of the radiation).

Production and Handling of Radiopharmaceuticals

The following paragraphs concern special considerations applying to the monographs on radiopharmaceuticals. The facilities for the production, use, and storage of radiopharmaceuticals are generally subject to licensing by national authorities. They often have to comply with 2 sets of regulations, those concerned with pharmaceutical preparations and those concerned with radioactive materials. Each producer or user must be thoroughly cognizant of the national requirements pertaining to the articles concerned.

Carriers

The mass of radioactive material usually encountered in radioactive pharmaceuticals is often too small to be measured by ordinary chemical or physical methods. Since such small amounts may not be subject to the usual methods of separation and purification, a *carrier*, in the form of inactive material, either isotopic with the radionuclide, or non-isotopic, but chemically similar to the radionuclide, may be added during processing and dispensing to permit ready handling. Thus sodium phosphate carrier is present in "Natrii Phosphatis (^{32}P) Injectio" and rhenium is used as a carrier in certain colloidal preparations of technetium-99m. The amount of carrier added must be sufficiently small for it not to cause undesirable physiological effects. The mass of an element formed in a nuclear reaction may be exceeded by that of the inactive isotope present in the target material or in the reagents used in the separation procedures.

Radioactive preparations in which no carrier is intentionally added during the manufacture or processing are often loosely referred to as *carrier-free*.

Detection and Measurement

Radioactive transformations may involve the emission of charged particles, the process of electron capture, or the process of isomeric transition. The charged particles emitted from the nucleus may be alpha-particles (helium nuclei of mass number 4) or beta particles (electrons of negative or positive charge, $\beta-$ or $\beta+$ respectively, the latter known as positrons). The emission of charged particles from the nucleus may be accompanied by gamma rays, which are of the same physical nature as X-rays. Gamma rays are also emitted in the process of isomeric transition (i.t.). X-rays, which may be accompanied by gamma rays, are emitted in the process of electron capture (e.c.). Positrons are annihilated on contact with matter. Each positron annihilated is accompanied by the emission of 2 gamma rays, each with an energy of 0.511 MeV.

The physical characteristics of radionuclides are summarized in Table 1.

The methods employed for the detection and measurement of radioactivity are dependent upon the nature and energy of the radiation emitted. Radioactivity may be detected and/or measured by a number of different instruments based upon the action of radiation in causing the ionization of gases and solids, or the fluorescence of certain solids and liquids, or by the effect of radiation on a photographic emulsion.

In general, a counting assembly consists of a sensing unit and an electronic scaling device. The sensing unit may be a Geiger-Müller tube, a proportional counter, a scintillation detector in which a photomultiplier tube is employed in conjunction with a scintillator, or a solid-state semiconductor.

Geiger-Müller counters and proportional counters are generally used for the measurement of the beta emitters. Scintillation counters

TABLE 1. PHYSICAL CHARACTERISTICS OF RADIONUCLIDES

Nuclide	Half-life period[a]	Type of decay[b]	Particle energies and transition probabilities		Electromagnetic transitions		
			energy MeV	transition probability	photon energy MeV	photons emitted	transitions internally converted
Cesium-137	30.1 a	β−	0.512 1.174	94.6 % 5.4 %	via 2.6 min 137mBa 0.662 0.032–0.038	85.1 % 8 % (Ba K X-rays)	9.5 %
Chromium-51	27.7 d	e.c.		100 %	0.320 0.005–0.006	9.83 % ~22 % (V K X-rays)	
Cobalt-57	270 d	e.c.		100 %	0.014 0.122 0.136 0.570 0.692 others 0.006–0.007	9.4 % 85.2 % 11.1 % 0.02 % 0.16 % low intensity ~55 % (Fe K X-rays)	78.0 % 2.0 % 1.5 %
Cobalt-58	70.8 d	β+ e.c.	0.475	15.0 % 85.0 %	0.511 0.811 0.864 1.675 0.006–0.007	from β+ 99.4 % 0.7 % 0.5 % ~26 % (Fe K X-rays)	

a μs = microsecond; ms = millisecond; s = second; min = minute; h = hour; d = day; a = year.
b e.c. = electron capture; i.t. = isomeric transition.

TABLE 1. PHYSICAL CHARACTERISTICS OF RADIONUCLIDES (continued)

Nuclide	Half-life period[a]	Type of decay[b]	Particle energies and transition probabilities		Electromagnetic transitions		
			energy MeV	transition probability	photon energy MeV	photons emitted	transitions internally converted
Cobalt-60	5.27 a	β−	0.318	99.9 %	1.173	99.86 %	0.02 %
			1.491	0.1 %	1.333	99.98 %	0.01 %
					others	<0.01 %	
Gallium-67	78.3 h	e.c.		100 %	0.091	3.6 %	0.3 %
					0.185	23.5 %	0.4 %
					0.209	2.6 %	0.02 %
					0.300	16.7 %	0.06 %
					0.394	4.4 %	0.01 %
					0.494	0.1 %	
					0.704	0.02 %	
					0.795	0.06 %	
					0.888	0.17 %	
					0.008–0.010	43 % (Zn K X-rays)	
					via 9.2 μs ^{67m}Zn		
					0.093	37.6 %	32.4 %
					0.008–0.010	13 % (Zn K X-rays)	
Gold-198	2.70 d	β−	0.285	1.32 %	0.412	95.45 %	4.3 %
			0.961	98.66 %	0.676	1.06 %	0.03 %
			1.373	0.02 %	1.088	0.23 %	
Gold-199	3.13 d	β−	0.25	21 %	0.050	0.3 %	3.5 %
			0.29	72 %	0.158	39.6 %	36.4 %
			0.45	7 %	0.208	8.8 %	8.3 %
					0.069–0.083	~18 % (Hg K X-rays)	

Nuclide	Half-life	Decay mode		Particle energy (MeV)	Photon energy (MeV)	Intensity	
Indium-111	2.81 d	e.c.	100 %		0.172 0.247	89.6 % 94.0 %	10.4 % 6.0 %
Indium-113m	99.5 min	i.t.	100 %		0.392 0.024–0.028	64.9 % (In K X-rays) 24 % (In K X-rays)	35.1 %
Iodine-123	13.2 h	e.c.	100 %		0.159 0.347 0.440 0.506 0.529 0.539 0.027–0.032	83.0 % 0.10 % 0.35 % 0.26 % 1.05 % 0.27 % ~86 % (Te K X-rays)	16.3 %
Iodine-125	60.0 d	e.c.	100 %		0.035 0.027–0.032	7 % 138 % (Te K X-rays)	93 %
Iodine-126	13 d	β- β+ e.c.	3 % 30 % 15 % ~0.1 % ~0.4 % 51.5 %	0.38 0.88 1.27 0.46 1.1	0.389 0.491 0.511 0.666 0.754 0.880 1.420 others 0.027–0.032	32 % 2 % from β+ 30 % 4 % 0.8 % 0.3 % <0.1 % each ~38 % (Te K X-rays)	0.5 % 0.1 %
Iodine-131	8.06 d	β-	1.8 % 0.6 % 7.2 % 89.7 % 0.7 %	0.247 0.304 0.334 0.606 0.806	0.080 0.284 0.364 0.637 0.723	2.4 % 5.9 % 81.8 % 7.2 % 1.8 %	3.8 % 0.3 % 1.7 %
						1.3 % of ^{131}I decays via 12 d ^{131m}Xe	
(Xenon-131m)		i.t.	100 %		0.164	2 %	98 %

(percentages relate to disintegrations of ^{131m}Xe)

a μs = microsecond; ms = millisecond; s = second; min = minute; h = hour; d = day; a = year.
b e.c. = electron capture; i.t. = isomeric transition.

TABLE 1. PHYSICAL CHARACTERISTICS OF RADIONUCLIDES (continued)

Nuclide	Half-life period[a]	Type of decay[b]	Particle energies and transition probabilities		Electromagnetic transitions		
			energy MeV	transition probability	photon energy MeV	photons emitted	transitions internally converted
Iodine-132	2.29 h	β−	0.84	16.0 %	0.506	5.0 %	
			1.01	3.5 %	0.523	16.1 %	0.2 %
			1.07	6.5 %	0.621	2.0 %	
			1.09	3.0 %	0.630	13.7 %	0.1 %
			1.10	2.6 %	0.651	2.7 %	
			1.26	2.9 %	0.668	98.7 %	0.4 %
			1.29	18.4 %	0.670	4.9 %	
			1.57	10.8 %	0.672	5.2 %	
			1.72	12.7 %	0.727	6.5 %	
			2.24	20.2 %	0.773	76.2 %	0.3 %
			others	3.4 %	0.810	2.9 %	
					0.812	5.6 %	
					0.955	18.1 %	
					1.136	3.0 %	
					1.295	2.0 %	
					1.372	2.5 %	
					1.399	7.1 %	
					1.433	1.4 %	
					1.921	1.2 %	
					2.002	1.1 %	
					others	< 1.5 %	
Iron-55	2.69 a	e.c.			0.006	~28 % (Mn K X-rays)	
Iron-59	44.6 d	β−	0.084	0.1 %	0.143	0.8 %	
			0.132	1.1 %	0.192	2.8 %	
			0.274	45.8 %	0.335	0.3 %	
			0.467	52.7 %	0.383	0.02 %	
			1.566	0.3 %	1.099	55.8 %	
					1.292	43.8 %	
					1.482	0.06 %	

Nuclide	Half-life	Decay mode[b]	Branching	Particle energy (MeV)	Photon energy (MeV)	Intensity	
Mercury-197	64.4 h	e.c.	100 %		0.077	19.2 %	80.7 %
					0.192	~1.1 %	0.9 %
					0.268	~0.1 %	
					0.067–0.080	~73 % (Au K X-rays)	
Mercury-197m	24 h	e.c.	6.5 %		0.134	31.8 %	61.7 %
		i.t.	93.5 %		0.165	0.3 %	93.2 %
					0.067–0.083	36 % (Au/Hg K X-rays)	
					via 7.8 s ^{197m}Au		
					0.130	0.5 %	6 %
					0.279	5.0 %	1.5 %
					0.409	<0.005 %	
					0.067–0.080	~2 % (Au K X-rays)	
Daughter ^{197}Hg							
Mercury-203	46.6 d	β−	100 %	0.212	0.279	81.5 %	18.5 %
					0.071–0.085	12.8 % (Tl K X-rays)	
Molybdenum-99	66.2 h	β−	18.3 %	0.454	0.041	1.2 %	4.8 %
			1.4 %	0.866	0.141	5.4 %	0.7 %
			80 %	1.232	0.181	6.6 %	1.0 %
			0.3 %	others	0.366	1.4 %	
					0.412	0.02 %	
					0.529	0.05 %	
					0.621	0.02 %	
					0.740	13.6 %	
					0.778	4.7 %	
					0.823	0.13 %	
					0.961	0.1 %	
					via 6.02 h ^{99m}Tc in equilibrium		
					0.002	~0 %	93.9 %
					0.141	83.9 %	10.0 %
					0.143	0.03 %	0.8 %

[a] μs = microsecond; ms = millisecond; s = second; min = minute; h = hour; d = day; a = year.
[b] e.c. = electron capture; i.t. = isomeric transition.

TABLE 1. PHYSICAL CHARACTERISTICS OF RADIONUCLIDES *(continued)*

Nuclide	Half-life period[a]	Type of decay[b]	Particle energies and transition probabilities		Electromagnetic transitions		
			energy MeV	transition probability	photon energy MeV	photons emitted	transitions internally converted
Phosphorus-32	14.3 d	β⁻	1.709	100 %			
Selenium-75	118.5 d	e.c.		100 %	0.066	1.1 %	
					0.097	2.9 %	0.3 %
					0.121	15.7 %	3.0 %
					0.136	54.0 %	0.7 %
					0.199	1.5 %	1.6 %
					0.265	56.9 %	
					0.280	18.5 %	0.4 %
					0.401	11.7 %	0.2 %
					others	<0.05 % each	
					0.010–0.012	~50 % (As K X-rays)	
					via 16.4 ms ⁷⁵mAs		
					0.024	0.03 %	5.5 %
					0.280	5.4 %	
					0.304	1.2 %	0.1 %
					0.010–0.012	~2.6 % (As K X-rays)	
	Daughter ⁹⁹Tc						
Technetium-99m	6.02 h	i.t.		100 %	0.002	~0 %	99.1 %
					0.141	88.5 %	10.6 %
					0.143	0.03 %	0.87 %
Thallium-201	73.5 h	e.c.		100 %	0.031	0.29 %	10.1 %
					0.032	0.25 %	9.6 %
					0.135	2.9 %	8.9 %
					0.166	0.13 %	0.2 %
					0.167	8.81 %	16.0 %

Radionuclide	Half-life	Decay mode	β energy (MeV)	%	Photon energy (MeV)	%	%
Tin-113	115 d	e.c.		100 %	0.255 / 0.024–0.028	2.1 % (In K X-rays) / 73 %	0.1 %
Daughter ^{113m}In							
Tritium (^{3}H)	12.35 a	β−	0.0186	100 %			
Xenon-131m	11.9 d	i.t.		100 %	0.164 / 0.029–0.035	2 % / ~52 % (Xe K X-rays)	98 %
Xenon-133	5.25 d	β−	0.266 / 0.346	0.9 % / 99.1 %	0.080 / 0.081 / 0.160 / 0.030–0.036	0.4 % / 36.6 % / 0.05 % / ~46 % (Cs K X-rays)	0.5 % / 63.3 %
Xenon-133m	2.26 d	i.t.		100 %	0.233 / 0.029–0.035	8 % / ~59 % (Xe K X-rays)	92 %
Daughter ^{133}Xe							
Ytterbium-169	32.0 d	e.c.		100 %	0.021 / 0.063 / 0.094 / 0.110 / 0.117 / 0.118 / 0.131 / 0.177 / 0.198 / 0.240 / 0.261 / 0.308	0.21 % / 45.16 % / 0.78 % / 3.82 % / 0.04 % / 1.90 % / 11.42 % / 17.31 % / 26.16 % / 0.12 % / 1.74 % / 11.04 %	12.3 % / 50.4 % / 12.3 % / 56.2 % / 3.2 % / 13.5 % / 17.7 % / 25.7 % / 0.7 %

[a] μs = microsecond; ms = millisecond; s = second; min = minute; h = hour; d = day; a = year.
[b] e.c. = electron capture; i.t. = isomeric transition.

employing liquid or solid phosphors may be used for the measurement of alpha, beta, and gamma emitters. Solid-state devices may also be used for alpha, beta, and gamma measurements. The electronic circuitry associated with a detector system usually consists of a high-voltage supply, an amplifier, a pulse-height selector, and a scaler, a ratemeter, or other readout device. When the electronic scaling device or the scaler in a counting assembly is replaced by an electronic integrating device, the resultant assembly is a ratemeter. Ratemeters are used for the purpose of monitoring and surveying radioactivity and are somewhat less precise as measuring instruments than the counters. Ionization chambers are often used for measuring gamma-ray activities and, provided they are thin-walled, for measuring X-rays.

Radiation from a radioactive source is emitted in all directions. Procedures for the standardization and measurement of such sources by means of a count of the emissions in all directions are known as 4π-counting; those based on a count of the emissions in a solid angle of 2π steradians are known as 2π-counting; and those based on a fraction of the emissions defined by the solid angle subtended from the detector to the source are known as counting in a fixed geometry. It is customary to assay the radioactivity of a preparation by comparison with a standardized preparation using identical geometry conditions. The validity of such an assay is critically dependent upon the reproducibility of the spatial relationships of the source to the detector and its surroundings and upon the accuracy of the standardized preparation. In the primary standardization of radionuclides coincidence techniques are employed in preference to simple 4π-counting whenever the decay scheme of the radionuclide permits. One of the most commonly employed coincidence techniques is 4π-beta/gamma coincidence counting, which is used for nuclides in which some or all of the disintegrations are followed by prompt photon emission. An additional adjacent detector, sensitive only to photons, is used to measure the efficiency in the 4π-counter of those disintegrations with which the photons are coincident. 4π-Gamma/gamma coincidence counting techniques are often employed for the standardization of pure gamma emitters.

The construction and performance of instruments and accessory apparatus vary. The preparation of samples must be modified to obtain satisfactory results with a particular instrument. The operator must follow carefully the manufacturer's instructions for optimum instrument performance and substantiate results by careful examination of known samples. Proper instrument functioning and reliability must be monitored on a day-to-day basis through the use of secondary reference preparations.

Radioactivity due to materials of construction, to cosmic rays, and to spontaneous discharges in the atmosphere contributes what is known as the *background activity*. All sample radioactivity measurements must be corrected by subtracting background activity.

In the counting of samples at high activity levels, corrections must be made also for loss of counts due to inability of the equipment to resolve pulses arriving in close succession. Such coincidence-loss corrections must be made prior to the subtraction of background correction.

The corrected count rate, R, is given by the formula

$$R = \frac{r}{1 - r\,\tau}$$

where r is the observed count rate, and τ is the resolving time.

A radioactivity count is a statistical value, i.e., it is a measure of nuclear decay probabilities, and is not exactly constant over any given time interval. The magnitude of the standard deviation is approximately equal to the square root of the number of counts. In general, at least 10 000 counts are necessary to obtain a standard deviation of 1 %.

Absorption

Ionizing radiation is absorbed in the material surrounding the source of the radiation. Such absorption occurs in air, in the sample itself (self-absorption), in sample coverings, in the window of the detection device, and in any special absorbers placed between the sample and the detector. Since alpha particles have a short range of penetration in matter, beta particles have a somewhat greater range, and gamma rays are deeply penetrating, identification of the type and energy of radiation emitted from a particular radionuclide may be determined by the use of absorbers of varying thickness. In practice, this method is little used, and then only in connexion with beta emitters. However, variations in counting rate due to variations in thickness and density of sample containers can be a major problem with beta emitters and with X-ray emitters, such a iodine-125. Plastic tubes, in which variations of density and thickness are minimal, are therefore often employed.

The absorption coefficient (μ), which is the reciprocal of the "thickness" expressed in mg/cm^2, or the half-thickness (the thickness of absorber required to reduce the radioactivity by a factor of two), is commonly determined to characterize the beta radiation emitted by a radionuclide.

Method

The following procedure is used for the identification test in "Natrii Phosphatis (^{32}P) Injectio" for the measurement of beta activity and for calculation of the absorption coefficient of half-thickness:

Place the radioactive substance, suitably mounted for counting, under a suitable counter. Make count rate determinations individually and successively, using at least 6 different thicknesses of aluminium foil chosen from a range of 10 to 200 mg/cm² and a single absorber with a thickness of at least 800 mg/cm². The sample and absorbers should be as close as possible to the detector in order to minimize scattering effects. Obtain the net beta count rate at the various absorbers used by subtracting the count rate found with the thickest absorber (800 mg/cm² or more). Plot the logarithm of the net beta count rate as a function of the total absorber thickness. The total absorber thickness is the thickness of the aluminium plus the thickness of the counter window (as stated by the manufacturer), plus the air-equivalent thickness (the distance, expressed in cm, of the sample from the counter window multiplied by 1.205), all expressed in mg/cm². An approximately straight line results.

Choose two of the absorber thicknesses (t_1 and t_2) that are 20 mg/cm² or more apart and that fall on the plot, and calculate the absorption coefficient (μ) from the equation

$$\mu = \frac{1}{t_2 - t_1} \ln \frac{A_{t_1}}{A_{t_2}}$$

where t_1 is the thinner absorber, t_2 is the thicker absorber, and A_{t_1} and A_{t_2} represent the net beta count rate with t_1 and t_2 absorbers, respectively. Alternatively the half-thickness may be read directly from the plot.

The choice of absorber thickness depends on the radionuclide. For radionuclides other than phosphorus-32, which have higher or lower beta energy, greater or lesser absorber thicknesses are necessary.

For characterization of the radionuclide, the absorption coefficient or the half-thickness should be within $\pm 5\,\%$ of that found for a sample of the same radionuclide of known purity when determined in parallel.

The count rate at zero total absorber thickness may be determined by plotting a curve identical with the one described for determination of the absorption coefficient and extrapolating the straight line plot to zero absorber thickness, taking into consideration the thickness, expressed in mg/cm², of sample coverings, the air, and the counter window.

Radiation spectrometry

Crystal scintillation spectrometry

When the energy of beta or gamma radiation is dissipated within materials known as scintillators, light is produced in an amount proportional to the energy dissipated. This quantity of light may be measured by suitable means, and is proportional to the energy absorbed in the scintillator. The light emitted under the impact of a gamma photon or a beta particle is converted into an electric output pulse by a photo-multiplier. Scanning of the output pulses with a suitable pulse-height analyser results in an energy spectrum of the source.

The scintillators most commonly used for gamma spectrometry are single crystals of thallium-activated sodium iodide. Gamma-ray scintillation spectra show one or more sharp, characteristic photoelectric peaks, corresponding to the energies of the gamma radiation of the source. They are thus useful for identification purposes and also for the detection of gamma-emitting impurities in a preparation. These peaks are accompanied by other peaks due to secondary effects of radiation on the scintillator and its surroundings, such as backscatter, positron annihilation, coincidence summing, and fluorescent X-rays. In addition, broad bands known as the Compton continua arise from the scattering of the gamma photons in the scintillator and in surrounding materials. Calibration of the instrument is achieved with the use of known samples of radionuclides whose energy spectra have been characterized. The shape of the spectrum produced will vary with the instrument used, owing to such factors as differences in the shape and size of the crystal, in the shielding materials used, the distance between the source and the detector, and in the types of discriminator employed in the pulse-height analysers. When using the spectrum for identification of radionuclides it is therefore necessary to compare the spectrum with that of a known sample of the radionuclide obtained in the same instrument under identical conditions.

Certain radionuclides, for example, iodine-125, emit characteristic X-rays of well-defined energies that will produce photoelectric peaks in a suitable gamma spectrometer. Beta radiation also interacts with the scintillators, but the spectra are continuous and diffuse and generally of no use for identification of the radionuclide or for the detection of beta-emitting impurities in a preparation.

Semiconductor detector spectrometry

Gamma-ray and beta-particle spectra may be obtained using solid-state detectors. The peaks obtained do not suffer to the same extent the broadening shown in crystal scintillation spectrometry, and the resolution of gamma photons of similar energies is very much improved. However, the efficiencies of such detectors are much lower.

The energy required to create an electron-hole pair or to promote an electron from the valence band to the conduction band in a semiconductor is far less than the energy required to produce a photon in a scintillation crystal. In gamma-ray spectrometry a lithium-drifted germanium detector can provide an energy resolution of 0.33 % for the 1.33 MeV photon of cobalt-60, as compared with 5.9 % with a 7.6-cm × 7.6-cm thallium-activated sodium iodide crystal.

Liquid scintillation counting

For weak beta-emitters like ^{35}S, ^{14}C and ^3H, where self-absorption of the low-energy beta particles is significant, the preferred counting method is by liquid scintillation, which can occasionally be employed also for emitters of X-rays, alpha-particles, and gamma-rays. If the sample to be counted is dissolved in, or mixed with, a solution of an appropriate scintillator material, the decay energy from the sample is converted into light photons. These are sensed by a photomultiplier, which converts them into an electric pulse, whose intensity is proportional to the energy of the initial radiation. Thus, simultaneous counting of several radionuclides differing in the energy of emitted radiation can be effected with suitable discriminators (pulse-height analysers), providing the energy separation is sufficient. Detection efficiencies approaching 95 % for ^{14}C and 60 % for ^3H are reached because self-absorption is minimized.

The scintillator solute usually consists of a polycyclic aromatic compound, such as *p*-terphenyl or 2,5-diphenyloxazole (primary solute), together with a secondary solute, such as 1,4-di[2-(4-methyl-5-phenyloxazole)]benzene (Dimethyl-POPOP), that shifts the wavelength of the light emitted to match the highest sensitivity of the photomultiplier tube. Water-immiscible solvents, such as toluene, or water-miscible solvents, such as dioxan, can be used. To facilitate the counting of aqueous solutions, special solvents have been developed. Alternatively, samples may be counted as suspensions in scintillator gels. As a means of attaining compatibility and miscibility with aqueous specimens to be assayed, many additives, such as surfactants and solubilizing agents, are also incorporated into the scintillator. For accurate determination of sample radioactivity, care must be exercised to prepare a sample that is truly homogeneous. The presence of impurities and colour in the solution causes a decrease in the number and energy of photons reaching the photomultiplier tube; such a decrease is known as quenching. Accurate radioactivity measurement requires correcting for count-rate loss due to quenching. Solutions containing organic scintillators are prone to photo-excitation and samples may need to be prepared in subdued light and kept in darkness before counting.

Radiation Shielding

Adequate shielding must be used to protect laboratory personnel from ionizing radiation, and measuring instruments must be suitably shielded from background radiation.

Alpha and beta radiations are readily shielded because of their limited range of penetration, although the production of *Bremsstrahlung* by the latter must be taken into account (see below). The range of alpha and beta particles varies inherently with their kinetic energy. The alpha particles are monoenergetic and have a range of a few centimetres in air. The absorption of beta particles, owing to their continuous energy spectrum and scattering, follows an approximately exponential function. The range of beta particles in air varies from centimetres to metres.

The secondary radiation produced by beta radiation upon absorption by shielding materials is known as *Bremsstrahlung* and resembles soft X-rays in its property of penetration. The higher the atomic number or density of the absorbing material, the greater the intensity of he *Bremsstrahlung* produced. Elements of low atomic number produce low-energy *Bremsstrahlung*, which is readily absorbed; therefore, materials of low atomic number or of low density, such as aluminium, glass, or transparent plastic, are used to shield sources of beta radiation.

Gamma-ray radiation is deeply penetrating. Attenuation of gamma-ray radiation in matter is exponential and is given in terms of half-value layers. The *half-value layer* is the thickness of shielding material necessary to decrease the intensity of radiation to half its initial value. A shield of 7 half-value layers is of a thickness that will reduce the intensity of radiation to less than 1 % of its unshielded intensity of activity. Gamma-ray radiation is commonly shielded with lead.

Intensity of gamma-ray radiation is diminished according to the inverse square of the intervening distance between the source and the point of reference. Radioactive materials of multimillicurie strength can be handled safely in the laboratory by using proper shielding and/or by arranging for the maximum practicable distance between the source and the operator by means of remote-handling devices.

Determination of Radionuclidic Purity

For gamma emitters the most useful method of examination for radionuclidic purity is gamma spectrometry. It is not, however, a completely certain method, because:

(*a*) beta-emitting impurities are, in general, not detected;

(*b*) when sodium iodide detectors are employed, the photoelectric peaks due to impurities may be obscured by those due to the major radionuclide, or, in other words, the degree of resolution of the instrument is insufficient; this problem can be overcome through the use of high resolution solid state semiconductor detectors, such as a lithium-drifted germanium (Ge:Li) detector;

(c) unless the instrument has been calibrated with a standard source of known radionuclidic purity under identical conditions of geometry, it is difficult to determine whether additional peaks are due to impurities or whether they result from such secondary effects as backscatter, coincidence summation, or fluorescent X-rays.

The range of gamma spectrometry may be extended in two ways: first, by observing changes in the spectrum of a preparation with time (this is especially useful in detecting the presence of long-lived impurities in a preparation of a short-lived radionuclide); secondly, by the use of chemical separations, whereby the major radionuclide may be removed by chemical means and the residue examined for impurities, or whereby specific impurities may be separated chemically and then quantified. It is evident that chemical means will not separate an impurity that is isotopic with the major radionuclide.

Requirements for radionuclidic purity

Requirements for radionuclidic purity are specified in two ways:

1. By expression of a minimum level of radionuclidic purity. Unless otherwise stated in the individual monograph, the gamma-ray spectrum, as determined by simple gamma spectrometry employing a sodium iodide detector, should not be significantly different from that of a standardized solution of the radionuclide before the expiry date is reached. As discussed above, it is difficult to set more precise requirements for a minimum level of radionuclidic purity.

2. By expression of maximum levels of specific radionuclidic impurities in the individual monographs. In general, such impurities are those that are known to be likely to arise during the production of the material — for example, mercury-203 in a preparation of mercury-197.

It is evident that while the above requirements are necessary, they are not in themselves sufficient to ensure that the radionuclidic purity of a preparation is sufficient for human use. A duty must remain with the manufacturer to examine his products in detail, and especially to examine preparations of short-lived radionuclides for long-lived impurities after a suitable period of decay. In this way, the manufacturer may satisfy himself that the manufacturing processes employed are producing materials of appropriate purity. In particular, the radionuclidic composition of certain preparations is determined by the chemical and isotopic composition of the target material, which is irradiated with neutrons, and trial preparations are advisable when new batches of target material are employed.

Determination of Radiochemical Purity

Radiochemical purity can be studied by a variety of techniques, but paper chromatography and thin-layer chromatography (see pp. 80-84) are of particular importance. After completion of the separation, the distribution of radioactivity on the chromatogram is determined. The weight of substance applied to the chromatogram is often extremely small (because of the great sensitivity of detection of the radioactivity) and particular care has to be taken in interpretation with regard to the formation of artefacts. Instead of chromatography, electrophoresis may be used for separation (see pp. 98-102). As mentioned above, the addition of carriers (i.e., the corresponding non-radioactive compounds) for both the radiopharmaceutical itself and the suspected impurities is sometimes helpful. There is, however, a danger that when an inactive carrier of the radiopharmaceutical is added it may interact with the radiochemical impurity, leading to underestimation of these impurities. Another useful technique involves monitoring the biological distribution of the injected radiopharmaceutical in suitable test animals.

Determination of Chemical Purity

Chemical purity refers to the proportion of the preparation that is in the specified chemical form regardless of the presence of radioactivity; it may be determined by normal methods of analysis.

The chemical purity of a preparation is often no guide to its radiochemical purity. Preparations, especially those resulting from exchange reactions (for example, a preparation of o-iodohippuric acid in which some of the iodine atoms are replaced by atoms of iodine-131), may be of high chemical purity but may contain impurities of high specific activity (that is, a tiny weight of an impurity may be associated with a relatively large amount of the radionuclide).

In general, chemical impurities in preparations of radiopharmaceuticals are objectionable only if they are toxic or if they modify the physiological processes that are under study.

Tests for Sterility and Pyrogens

A number of monographs for radiopharmaceuticals contain the requirement that the product be sterile and free of pyrogens. The half-life of radiopharmaceutical products is such that, as a rule only tests for pyrogens can be completed prior to release. Tests for sterility must, in general, be completed retrospectively.

Sterility tests

The manufacturer should begin the sterility test as soon as possible and read the results after release.

A particular responsibility falls upon the manufacturer of radiopharmaceuticals to validate the sterilization process by all suitable measures, which may include careful and frequent calibration of sterilizers and the use of biological and chemical indicators of the efficiency of the sterilization process.

Pyrogen tests

The manufacturer also bears a particular responsibility to ensure that all substances used in the preparation of radiopharmaceuticals are handled in a manner that ensures their freedom from pyrogens. Pyrogen tests are specified in certain monographs where there are special dangers (see also pp. 155-156).

Addition of Bacteriostatic Agents

Injections of radiopharmaceuticals are commonly supplied in containers that are sealed to permit the withdrawal of successive doses on different occasions. The *International Pharmacopoeia* normally requires that such injections should contain a suitable bacteriostatic agent in a suitable concentration.

Many common bacteriostatic agents (for example, benzyl alcohol) are gradually destroyed by the effect of radiation in aqueous solutions. The rate of destruction is dependent upon a number of factors, including the nature of the radionuclide and the radioactive concentration of the solution. It is therefore not always possible to prescribe an effective bacteriostatic agent for an injection of a radiopharmaceutical and for certain preparations the addition of an agent is undesirable; for this reason the inclusion of bacteriostatic agents is not mandatory. The nature of the bacteriostatic agent, if present, must be stated on the label; if no bacteriostatic agent is present, this must also be stated. Radiopharmaceuticals whose expiry periods are greater than one day and that do not contain a bacteriostatic agent should preferably be supplied in single-dose containers.

Other Requirements

Radiopharmaceuticals administered parenterally should comply with the relevant requirements for injections in the *International Pharmacopoeia*, except that they are not subject to the requirements concerning volume of injection in a single-dose container.

Expiry Date

The special nature of a radiopharmaceutical requires that it be assigned an expiry period (or an expiry date), beyond which its continued use is not recommended. The expiry period so designated begins with the date at which the radioactivity is expressed on the label, and may be stated in terms of days, weeks or months. For longer-lived radionuclides, the expiry period does not exceed 6 months. The expiry period depends on the radiochemical stability and the content of longer-lived radionuclidic impurity in the preparation under consideration. At the end of the expiry period, the radioactivity will have decreased to the extent where insufficient radioactivity remains to serve the intended purpose or where the dose of active ingredient must be increased so much that undesirable physiological responses occur. In addition, chemical or radiation decomposition may have reduced the radiochemical purity to an unacceptable extent. Also the radionuclidic impurity content may be such that an unacceptable radiation dose would be delivered to the patient. The use of products beyond their expiry periods is therefore inadvisable.

Labelling

In general, the following information should appear on the immediate container (for example, vial):

(1) the name of the preparation;

(2) a statement that the product is radioactive;

(3) the name and location of the manufacturer;

(4) the total radioactivity present at a stated date and hour (whenever the half-life period is more than 30 days only the date need be stated);

(5) the expiry date or the expiry period;

(6) a number or other indication by which the history of the product may be traced (for example, batch or lot number);

(7) in the case of solutions, the total volume of the solution;

(8) special storage requirements with respect to temperature and light.

NOTE : In the case of a solution, instead of a statement of the total radioactivity, a statement of the radioactive concentration (for example, in mCi or MBq per ml of the solution) may be given.

The shipment of radioactive substances is subject to special national and international regulations as regards their packaging and outer labelling.

Storage

Radiopharmaceuticals should be kept in well-closed containers and stored in an area assigned for the purpose. The storage conditions should be such that the maximum radiation dose rate to which persons may be exposed is reduced to an acceptable level. Care should be taken to comply with national regulations for protection against ionizing radiation. Glass containers may darken under the effect of radiation.

POWDER FINENESS AND SIEVES

A. Powders

The degree of coarseness or fineness of a powder is differentiated by the nominal aperture size of the mesh of the sieve through which the powder is able to pass, expressed in μm.

The following terms are used in the description of powders:

Coarse powder (2000/355). A powder of which all the particles pass through a No. 2000 sieve, and not more than 40 % through a No. 355 sieve.

Moderately coarse powder (710/250). A powder of which all the particles pass through a No. 710 sieve, and not more than 40 % through a No. 250 sieve.

Moderately fine powder (355/180). . A powder of which all the particles pass through a No. 355 sieve, and not more than 40 % through a No. 180 sieve.

Fine powder (180). A powder of which all the particles pass through a No. 180 sieve.

Very fine powder (125). A powder of which all the particles pass through a No. 125 sieve.

When the fineness of a powder is described by means of a number, it is intended that all the particles of the powder should pass through the sieve distinguished by that number.

B. Sieves

The wire sieves used in sifting powdered drugs are distinguished by numbers, which indicate the nominal aperture size expressed in μm.

The sieves are made of wires of uniform circular cross-section, in accordance with the specifications given in Table 2.

TABLE 2. WIRE MESH SIEVES

Number of sieve (μm)	Nominal size of aperture (mm)	Nominal diameter of wire (mm)	Approximate screening area (%)
2000	2.00	0.90	48
710	0.710	0.450	37
500	0.500	0.315	38
355	0.355	0.224	38
250	0.250	0.160	37
212	0.212	0.140	36
180	0.180	0.125	35
150	0.150	0.100	36
125	0.125	0.090	34
90	0.090	0.063	35
75	0.075	0.050	36
45	0.045	0.032	34

The nominal size of aperture of wire mesh sieves has been selected principally from among those recommended in the ISO standard 565-1972.

PHYSICOCHEMICAL METHODS

CHROMATOGRAPHY

Chromatographic processes involve, in general, the distribution of a solute between two phases, one of which is the mobile phase and the other the stationary phase. The stationary phase may act by adsorption, by partition (where, for example, a liquid that is immiscible with the mobile phase may be coated on the surface of a solid support), by ion exchange, or by gel permeation. In practice, the chromatographic process in many pharmaceutical applications may be a complex synthesis of several physical phenomena; certainly many chromatographic procedures that are referred to as partition methods may be significantly influenced by adsorption effects.

Chromatography is thus simply a method of separation and of itself does not permit either identification or quantitative measurement. It is the combination of chromatography with appropriate methods of detection and measurement that results in the loosely but conveniently termed "chromatographic method of analysis".

For convenience the types of chromatography that are useful in pharmaceutical analysis may be considered as falling into three broad groups. In the planar methods, chromatography is effected by allowing the mobile phase to flow over and through a layer of the adsorbent (paper and thin-layer chromatography). In column methods, the adsorbent is packed into a column, which may be of the traditional open type or may be closed and designed to withstand considerable pressures so that the mobile phase may be pumped through the column at high speed (high-pressure liquid chromatography — sometimes known as high-performance or high-speed liquid chromatography). Gas chromatography is a special case of column chromatography in that the mobile phase is a gas rather than a liquid and the solutes must be volatile or rendered so by elevated temperatures and/or by conversion to volatile derivatives.

No one method of chromatography is adequate for all purposes, since each has its advantages and disadvantages. Most of the planar methods are simple and effective and require inexpensive equipment (although some complex accessories are available); these methods are valuable for identification and screening purposes but are less suitable for precise quantitative applications. Older column methods may be used without great expense but are often time-consuming and tedious to carry out. High-pressure liquid and gas chromatographic methods need specialized apparatus but may afford rapid and effective separations that are suitable for precise quantitative measurement of components.

Such methods are particularly valuable for the determination of small amounts of impurities. Limitations are currently imposed on the value of high-pressure liquid chromatography by the lack of universally applicable methods of detection and on that of gas-liquid chromatography by the non-volatility or thermal instability of many compounds.

Thin-layer Chromatography

In thin-layer chromatography the adsorbent is a thin, uniform layer (usually about 0.24 mm thick) of a dry, finely powdered material applied to a suitable support, such as a glass plate or an aluminium or plastic foil. The mobile phase is allowed to move across the surface of the plate (usually by capillary action) and the chromatographic process may depend upon adsorption, partition, or a combination of both, depending on the adsorbent, its treatment, and the nature of the solvents used. During the chromatographic procedure the plate is contained in a chromatographic chamber (usually made of glass to permit observation of the movement of the mobile phase up the plate), which is usually saturated with the solvent vapour. Solid supports frequently used are silica gel, kieselguhr, alumina, and cellulose; to these may be added suitable substances, for example, calcium sulfate to promote adhesion to the support. The prepared layer may be impregnated with buffering materials to afford acidic, neutral, or basic layers, or with other material, such as silver nitrate, designed to modify its properties. In certain cases the layer may consist of an ion-exchange material. This wide range of possible layers, used in conjunction with different solvent systems allows an almost infinite variation of separating power that makes thin-layer chromatography such a useful technique in pharmaceutical analysis.

As an adjunct to identification, thin-layer chromatography may be used by comparing the behaviour of the material to be identified with that of a standard substance, usually an authentic specimen of the substance being examined. If the two substances move identical distances during the chromatographic process and if the two substances, when mixed together and then subjected to chromatography, move as a single substance, it may be presumed that the two substances are identical. This presumption may be strengthened by repeating the procedure using a different system of chromatography; in general, if two substances behave identically in as many as three fundamentally different systems the presumption of identity becomes very strong.

For identification purposes it it convenient to define the relative distance that the unknown material moves in relation to the distance moved either by the solvent front or by a standard reference material. On a developed chromatogram, the ratio of the distance travelled on the adsorbent by a given compound to that travelled by the leading edge oft he solvent (or mobile phase), both measured from the point of application of the test substance, is referred to as the R_f value of the substance in the given chromatographic system. The ratio of the distances moved by the compound and a stated reference susbtance is referred to as the R_r value. In practice R_f values may vary considerably according to the exact experimental conditions so that the R_r value determined against the reference substance subjected to chromatography on the same surface gives a more reliable numerical value. Even more reliable, however, is comparison with an authentic specimen as described above and this is the procedure usually used for pharmacopoeial purposes.

To determine the position of a colourless substance on a developed chromatogram it is usually necessary to treat the chromatogram with a reagent that will either char the separated substances or convert them to coloured or fluorescent derivatives. A convenient alternative that is frequently applicable is to carry out the chromatography on a surface impregnated with a substance that fluoresces strongly when examined under short-wave ultraviolet light. Areas of the plate occupied by substances absorbing at the same wavelengthshow as dark spots on the fluorescent background. In special cases, other means of recognition may be used, for example, the detection of radioactivity where labelled compounds are being separated or a microbiological response where antibiotics are concerned.

The most valuable use of thin-layer chromatography in pharmaceutical work is to provide a means of assessing low levels of impurities in medicinal substances. For this purpose the substance is applied to the chromatographic surface and, after chromatography, any secondary spots to be seen in the chromatogram after appropriate visualization are compared for size and intensity with those of low loadings of expected impurities that have simultaneously been subjected to chromatography on the same plate. Such a procedure requires that the expected impurities be available and in certain monographs the use of authentic specimens of impurities is called for. Frequently, such impurities are not available and in such cases it is often possible to compare secondary spots arising from trace impurities with the spot obtained by carrying out chromatography on the same plate using an appropriately low loading of the substance being examined. This expedient is not always possible since impurities and the substance being examined may respond in different ways to the method of revelation used, but it often provides an acceptable criterion by which the level of impurity in the substance may be judged. A third procedure that is sometimes advocated is to apply such an amount of the substance being examined that, after chromatography, no secondary spots will appear if the sample is acceptably pure. This is the least satisfactory of the three methods since ability to see a secondary spot is a subjective matter and because the intensity of spots on a chromatogram may vary considerably from one occasion to another depending on the exact conditions of chromatography.

For quantitative procedures the spot may be removed from the plate, the substance eluted with a suitable solvent and then determined by a sufficiently sensitive method, such as a spectrophotometric measurement, either directly or after a chemical reaction. In certain cases, quantitation can also be achieved by measurement of the spot intensity with the aid of a scanning densitometer and subsequent comparison of the intensity with the intensities obtained from standard amounts of the same substance similarly treated.

Separations effected by thin-layer chromatography may sometimes be improved by multiple development (when the chromatogram is allowed to dry and then subjected again to the same system of chromatography), by continuous development (when the mobile phase is allowed to evaporate continuously from the upper end of the adsorbent surface), or by two-dimensional chromatography (when the chromatographic plate is allowed to dry, turned at right angles, and then subjected to further chromatography, frequently in a different solvent system from that used for the initial chromatography). Caution should be exercised in interpreting the results of chromatograms where such intermediate drying processes are used, however, since decomposition, such as oxidation, of the substance being chromatographed may occur on the plate. The process of two-dimensional chromatography is especially valuable in judging whether any chemical change is taking place during the development process. If a mixture of substances is developed first in one direction and then at right angles with the same solvent the separated substances will lie in a diagonal line across the plate if no artefacts are being produced.

In thin-layer chromatography the adsorbent is usually spread in a thin even layer on a support plate. This may be undertaken in the analytical laboratory but it is also possible and convenient to obtain commercially prepared chromatographic surfaces that are attached to glass or to plastic or metal foil. Unfortunately, so sensitive may the chromatographic process be to minor changes in conditions that these various commercially available materials are not always interchangeable one with another or with an apparently similar laboratory-coated plate. A factory-coated silica gel plate prepared by a given manufacturer may give different separation characteristics from a laboratory-coated plate prepared using the same manufacturer's coating substance, and instances exist where a perfectly satisfactory method of separation devised using laboratory-prepared plates fails when using precoated plates and vice versa. Great caution must therefore be exercised when changing from one type of chromatographic plate to another and the suitability of a given type of plate should always be assessed before reliance is placed upon it.

The chromatographic chamber in which chromatography takes place should be protected from light if it is suspected that the materials to be examined may be unstable in light. In any case, the chromatographic chamber should always be in a position where the direct rays of the sun cannot fall on it since the rays may be refracted to different degrees owing to imperfections in the glass walls of the chamber. This may give rise to areas of elevated temperature on the chromatographic plate and result in erratic flow of the mobile phase.

RECOMMENDED PROCEDURE

The method given below assumes the use of a laboratory-prepared chromatographic plate but a precoated plate, activated if necessary, may be used provided that it has been shown to be suitable for the particular application.

The equipment consists of:

• a device for spreading on plates a uniform layer of coating substance of the desired thickness;

• plates 200 mm long and wide enough to accommodate the required number of solutions to be examined and the reference solutions;

• a chromatographic chamber of transparent material, usually glass, with a tightly fitting lid, of a size suitable for the plates used.

Prepare a slurry of the coating substance and, using the spreading device, coat the carefully cleaned plates with a layer about 0.25 mm thick, unless otherwise specified in the monograph. Allow the coated plates to dry in air and heat to activate, unless otherwise specified in the monograph, at 110 °C for 30 minutes, then allow to cool. If the plates are not to be used immediately, store them in a desiccator containing silica gel, desiccant, R. Remove a narrow strip (2–5 mm) of the coating substance from the vertical sides of the plate.

Unless otherwise specified in the monograph, work under saturated chamber conditions. To achieve such conditions, line the chromatographic chamber with filter-paper and pour into the chamber a sufficient quantity of the mobile phase to saturate the filter-paper and form a layer about 5 mm deep. Close the chamber and allow to stand for at least 1 hour at room temperature.

Method

All operations during which the plate is exposed to the air should preferably be carried out at a relative humidity of 50–60 %. Apply the volume of the solution as specified in the monograph as a compact spot, preferably not more than 4 mm in diameter. Application may be made using a micropipette, a syringe, or other suitable means. The spot should be placed about 1.5 cm from the lower edge and not less than 2 cm from the vertical sides of the plate. Where more than one chromatogram is run on the same plate, the spots should be placed not less than 1.5 cm apart and form a line parallel with the lower edge of the plate. When the solvent has evaporated, place the plate in the chromatographic chamber, ensuring that the plate is as nearly vertical as possible and that the starting points are above the level of the mobile phase. Close the chamber and maintain it at a constant temperature. Allow the mobile phase to ascend the prescribed distance, usually 10–15 cm, remove the plate, mark the position of the solvent front and dry as specified in the monograph.

Paper Chromatography

In paper chromatography the stationary phase is a sheet of paper of suitable texture and thickness, which may sometimes be impregnated with a liquid phase that is immiscible with the mobile phase.

Chromatographic separations on paper are usually considerably slower than on thin-layer plates and the method is, in general, not so versatile as thin-layer chromatography since the degree of variation of the stationary phase is much more restricted. Neither is it possible to use the variety of corrosive detection reagents that is commonly employed when the adsorbent is an inorganic material coated on a glass plate. Nevertheless, paper chromatography is still a useful technique and certain very effective separations that were originally devised using paper have never been successfully transferred to the thin-layer plate. For semi-quantitative and quantitative work it is considerably easier and more effective to cut out a required area of paper and to elute a separated component than it is to remove completely the powder layer for elution, as is necessary with thin-layer chromatography.

The concepts of R_f and R_r values referred to in the discussion on thin-layer chromatography apply equally well to paper chromatography. Because of the nature of the adsorbent it is possible to carry out paper chromatography in either a descending or an ascending mode.

RECOMMENDED PROCEDURE

Descending paper chromatography

The apparatus consists of a glass chamber of suitable dimensions to accommodate the chromatographic paper used, ground at the top to take a closely fitting glass lid. The lid has a central hole about 1.5 cm in diameter closed by a heavy glass rod or a stopper. In the upper part of the chamber is suspended a solvent trough with a device, usually a glass rod, for holding the chromatographic paper. On either side of the trough, parallel to and slightly above its upper edges, are two glass guide rods to support the paper in such a manner that no part of it is in contact with the walls of the chamber. The chromatographic paper consists of suitable filter-paper, cut into strips of sufficient length, and of any convenient width between 2.5 cm and the length of the trough; the paper is cut so that the mobile phase runs in the direction of the grain of the paper.

Method

Place in the bottom of the chromatographic chamber a layer 2–3 cm deep of the stationary phase specified in the monograph. Close the chamber, and allow to stand for 24 hours at constant temperature. All operations during which the paper is exposed to the air should preferably be carried out at a relative humidity of about 50 %. Maintain the chamber under these conditions throughout the subsequent procedure. Draw a fine pencil line horizontally across the paper at such a distance from one end that when this end is secured in the solvent trough and the remainder of the paper is hanging freely over the guide rod the line is a few centimetres below the guide rod and parallel to it. Using a micropipette, syringe, or other suitable means, apply to a spot on the pencil line the volume of the solution specified in the monograph. If the total volume to be applied would produce a spot more than 10 mm in diameter, apply the solution in portions, allowing each to dry before the next application. When more than one chromatogram is to be run on the same strip of paper, space the solutions along the pencil line at points not less than 3 cm apart. Insert the paper in the chamber, close the lid, and allow to stand for 90 minutes. Introduce into the solvent trough, through the hole in the lid, a sufficient quantity of the mobile phase specified in the monograph, close the chamber and allow development to proceed for the prescribed distance or time. Remove the paper from the chromatographic chamber and allow to dry in air. The paper should be protected from bright light during the development and drying processes.

Ascending paper chromatography

The apparatus consists of a glass chamber of suitable dimensions to accommodate the chromatographic paper used, ground at the top to take a closely fitting glass lid. In the top of the chamber is a device that suspends the chromatographic paper and is capable of being lowered without opening the chamber. In the bottom of the chamber is a dish to contain the mobile phase into which the paper may be lowered. The chromatographic paper consists of suitable filter-paper, cut into strips of sufficient length and not less than 2.5 cm wide; the paper is cut so that the mobile phase runs in the direction of the grain of the paper.

Method

Place in the dish a layer 2–3 cm deep of the mobile phase specified in the monograph. If specified in the monograph, pour the stationary phase between the walls of the chamber and the dish. Close the chromatographic chamber and allow to stand for 24 hours at constant temperature. Maintain the chamber at this temperature throughout the subsequent procedure. All operations during which the paper is exposed to the air should preferably be carried out at a relative humidity of about 50 %. Draw a fine pencil line horizontally across the paper 3 cm from one end. Using a micropipette, syringe, or other suitable means, apply to a spot on the pencil line the volume of the solution specified in the monograph. If the total volume to be applied would produce a spot more than 10 mm in diameter apply the solution in portions, allowing each to dry before the next application. When more than one chromatogram is to be run on the same strip of paper, space the solutions along the pencil line at points not less than 3 cm apart. Insert the paper into the chamber, close the lid, and allow to stand for 90 minutes. Lower the paper into the mobile phase specified in the monograph, and allow development to proceed for the prescribed distance or time. Remove the paper from the chamber and allow to dry in air. The paper should be protected from bright light during the development and drying processes.

Column Chromatography

In *adsorption column chromatography* the solid support (e.g., activated alumina, powdered cellulose, silicic acid, or kieselguhr) is packed as a dry solid or as a slurry into a tube (glass, plastic, or other suitable material) having a restricted orifice (usually protected by a sintered glass disc) for efflux of the mobile phase. A solution of the material to be subjected to chromatography is added to the top of the column and allowed to flow into the adsorbent; the solvent that constitutes the mobile phase is then introduced in the top of the column and allowed to flow downwards either by gravity or by application of positive pressure; during this procedure care should be taken to ensure that the top of the column does not become dry. The effluent solution (known as the eluate) is monitored in either a continuous fashion (for example, with a flow-through ultraviolet absorption cell) or a stepwise fashion (for example, by collection of fractions at intervals determined by time or by volume or weight of eluate and subsequent examination of each fraction for the separated component). The need to examine individually many fractions in order to obtain a completely quantitative assessment of a substance has resulted in a decline in the use of classical column chromatographic procedures in recent years; where they do continue to be used, there is a natural tendency to favour methods of detection and determination that are readily adaptable to automated processes.

In *partition column chromatography*, a liquid stationary phase, which should be substantially immiscible with the mobile phase, is adsorbed to the surface of the solid adsorbent. Chromatography is carried out as described for adsorption column chromatography, the mobile phase being saturated with the stationary phase before it is used for elution. Usually the solid adsorbent in partition chromatography is polar and the adsorbed stationary phase is also polar with respect to the mobile phase. The most widely used adsorbent in this connexion is a siliceous earth having an appropriate particle size to permit ready flow of the mobile phase. In certain cases *reverse-phase* partition chromatography is useful; in this case the polar adsorbent is rendered non-polar by silanizing or other means, such as treatment with paraffins, and the adsorbed stationary phase is less polar than the mobile phase.

In these partition systems the degree of partition of a compound is governed by its distribution coefficient between the two liquid phases and, in the case of compounds that dissociate, by the pH of the more polar of the two phases. Selective elution of components of a mixture can often be achieved by successive changes in the mobile phase or by changing the pH of the stationary phase by using a mobile phase consisting of a solution of an appropriate acid or base in an organic solvent.

Ion-exchange chromatography may be considered a case of chromatography where the solid phase contains an ion-exchange material, usually called ion-exchange resin.

Ion-exchange is defined as the reversible interchange between the ion present in the solution and the counter-ion of the resinous polymer, modified cellulose, or bonded silica gel support; it may be exemplified for the H^+/Na^+ exchange of a strongly acidic cation-exchange resin as:

$$RSO_3H + Na^+ \rightleftharpoons RSO_3Na + H^+$$

and for a Cl^-/OH^- strongly basic anion-exchange resin as:

$$R'N(CH_3)_3OH + Cl^- \rightleftharpoons R'N(CH_3)_3Cl + OH^-$$

The selection of strong or weak resins, of either type, will largely depend on the pH at which the exchange is to be carried out and on the types of cation or anion that are to be exchanged. However, the strongly acidic and basic exchange resins will serve in most analytical applications.

Their specific capacity may vary from 2 to 5 millimoles per gram (dry basis). In practice, a large (200-300 %) excess of resin is used over the calculated stoichiometric requirement.

The laws governing the exchange reaction are complex, being in part described by mass action, ionic charge, and activity relationships. The selectivity coefficient is used to indicate the preference of the ion-exchange resin for the uptake of 2 (or more) ions from solution. Generally speaking, the resin will take up divalent (or higher) ions in preference to monovalent ions, and in the case of a choice between ions of the same valence, the resin will take up the heavier ion preferentially.

Treatment of the ion-exchange resin and preparation of the column. Usually the ion-exchange resin is immersed in water and allowed to swell for 24 hours; it is then packed into a suitable column and, in the case of an anion-exchange resin, converted to the basic form by passing sodium hydroxide ($\sim$80 g/l) TS through the column at a rate of about 3 ml per minute until the effluent is free of chloride, followed by carbon-dioxide-free water, R to remove alkalinity. In the case of a cation-exchange resin, conversion to the acidic form is achieved by passing hydrochloric acid ($\sim$70 g/l) TS through the column, followed by carbon-dioxide-free water R until the washings are neutral.

The prepared column is used in a similar manner to that described for adsorption column chromatography except that there is usually no need to monitor the effluent; according to the type of resin chosen and the type of material being determined the volume of effluent detailed in the particular application is collected and titrated with acid or base as appropriate, using a suitable indicator.

After the determination has been completed, the ion-exchange column may be regenerated by washing either with sodium hydroxide ($\sim$80 g/l) TS, for an anion-exchange column, or hydrochloric acid ($\sim$70 g/l) TS, for a cation-exchange column, followed by water until a neutral reaction is obtained.

High-pressure Liquid Chromatography

This most recently introduced method of chromatography has brought column chromatography, the oldest form of the art, back into prominence. The essential development that has made the technique possible has been the availability of highly pressure-resistant particles of uniform diameters of less than 50 μm. These particles commonly have a solid centre, for example, of glass, and a thin porous outer layer, for example, of silica; the small particle size and high surface area so obtained confer a very high efficiency for use in adsorption chromatography. When these particles are coated with a suitable stationary phase, high-pressure liquid chromatography may be used as a partition technique.

To ensure stability of the prepared column the stationary phases are frequently chemically bonded (usually by an ester or an ether linkage) to the support.   The ether bond affords a more stable product than the ester bond, which may be hydrolysed by polar solvents; for example, in octadecylsilane-coated beads the hydrocarbon chain is bonded by an ether linkage to glass beads coated with a thin layer of silica and these provide a very efficient reverse phase system that is highly stable in use. For chromatography, these particles are packed into narrow-bore (usually 2–4 mm internal diameter) columns; it is clear that such fine material packed into columns that may be up to 1 m in length will provide considerable resistance to the flow of the mobile phase and it is for this reason that high pressures must be employed.   Typical lengths of columns are 20–30 cm and conditions for quantitative analysis might be a flow rate of about 1–3 ml per minute and a pressure of up to 28 000 kPa (4 000 lbf/in^2).

More recently silica beads having a uniform diameter of about 5 μm have become available; they are porous throughout and may have surface areas as high as 300 m^2/g.   Consequently they give more effective separations than the 30–50 μm packing.   For column preparation it is possible to dry pack the larger particles, but for the 5 μm diameter material it is essential to use a slurrying technique.

In addition to the adsorption and partition modes referred to above, the principle of the high-pressure technique is applicable to ion-exchange chromatography provided that suitable resins are available as sufficiently small pressure-resistant particles.

With such high pressures it is obvious that specialized equipment is necessary.   The essential features of the apparatus are a suitable pump to deliver the mobile phase from an enclosed solvent reservoir to the column, a means of introducing the test solution on to the column (usually a form of injection valve designed to work at high pressure), the column itself (often at ambient temperature but sometimes maintained at temperatures up to 100 °C), an appropriate detector system, and an amplifier connected to a suitable recording device, such as a strip-chart recorder, where signals may be plotted against time, or an electronic integrator.

As detectors, the most commonly employed at the present stage of development of the method are the ones based on ultraviolet spectrophotometry or on measurements of refractive index or on fluorescence measurements.   For pharmaceutical work, the ultraviolet spectrophotometer is the most suitable because of its sensitivity (the lower limit of detectability may be of the order of 1 or 2 ng for materials having good light absorbing properties) and its stability (particularly its low sensitivity to controlled changes in solvent composition and flow irregularities); naturally, such a detector fails completely when materials exhibiting no significant absorption in ultraviolet light are eluted.   The refractometer responds to differences in refractive index between the pure mobile phase and mobile phase containing an eluted material; it is a more generally applicable method than ultraviolet absorption spectrophotometry but lacks sensitivity and is seriously affected by small changes in solvent composition, flow rate, and temperature.

For some applications, particularly in experiments designed to determine optimum solvent composition for a method that is subsequently to be used in a routine fashion, the technique of gradient elution is useful. The composition of the solvent mixture constituting the mobile phase is continuously varied at a predetermined rate during chromatography and this enables a single chromatogram to deal with complex mixtures of substances having greatly differing partition coefficients (the partition coefficient, K, as under gas chromatography (see below), being a measure of the amount of solute in the stationary phase compared to that in the mobile phase).

By using methods of computation similar to those referred to under gas chromatography, the high-pressure technique is capable of high precision and is thus very suitable for quantitative purposes. It is a rapid procedure and has been used to effect many highly efficient separations. It requires highly specialized apparatus, however, and, for many applications, expensive column packing materials. A potential advantage over gas chromatography is that volatility and thermostability, so important in gas chromatography, are of no concern. A disadvantage at the present time is that no universally applicable detector system is yet available.

Gas Chromatography

Gas chromatography may be regarded as a form of column chromatography in which the mobile phase is a gas (referred to as the carrier gas) rather than a liquid solvent. The stationary phase may be an active adsorbent such as alumina, silica gel, or carbon (gas-solid chromatography) or it may be a liquid that is coated as a thin film on a finely divided inert solid support such as diatomaceous earth, firebrick, glass beads, or other suitable material (gas-liquid chromatography); if the chromatographic column is of very small diameter the stationary phase may be coated on its inner wall to provide the so-called "open tube" or "capillary" column. Certain materials are available that do not require coating with a liquid phase, for example, polyaromatic porous beads, and these are of great value for specific applications.

The substance is introduced in a vaporized state into the carrier gas stream at the head of the column and it undergoes distribution between the gas and liquid or solid stationary phase in a similar manner to that in other forms of chromatography. The partition coefficient (K), which is defined as

$$K = \frac{\text{quantity of solute in the stationary phase}}{\text{quantity of solute in the mobile phase}},$$

will depend upon the nature of the solute, the nature and amount of the stationary phase, the temperature, and the carrier gas flow rate. It will be clear then that the value of K will depend upon the particular column and precise operating conditions used and, since these would be impossible to reproduce exactly from one laboratory to another and from one make of instrument to another, it is necessary to treat the operating conditions set down for pharmacopoeial purposes with a degree of flexibility that is not accorded to other, nonchromatographic, test procedures.

The essential features of the apparatus for effecting gas-liquid chromatography (much more widely used for pharmaceutical applications than adsorption chromatography on a solid) are a source of carrier gas (usually contained in compressed form in a cylinder fitted with a pressure-reducing valve), a flowmeter through which the gas passes, and an injection port that may be heated to a suitable temperature to volatilize but not decompose the substance and through which the test solution is introduced into the flow of carrier gas, preferably directly into the column packing. The constant flow of carrier gas is then maintained as the chromatographic process takes place, the components of the test solution being separated according to the value of K for each under the particular conditions being used.

As the components emerge from the column they enter a suitable differential-type detector, which usually depends on changes of ionization in a flame or on changes of thermal conductivity. Many other types of detectors exist and some of these are useful for specific pharmaceutical applications, for example, the electron capture detector that is of special value in the sensitive detection of halogenated compounds. Electrical signals from the detector are passed to an amplifier connected to a suitable recording device, such as a strip-chart recorder, where signals may be plotted against time. A powerful though very expensive means of detection is to use a mass spectrometer coupled to the gas chromatograph. This is very sensitive and provides information that enables unambiguous identification of substances issuing from the column.

The column is made of glass or metal (in the latter case care has to be taken since certain organic substances undergo metal-catalysed degradation reactions at elevated temperatures) and is contained in a temperature-controlled oven capable of being maintained at temperatures ranging from just above ambient temperature to about 300 °C according to the particular application. Ovens may also be controlled in such a way that a steady rise of temperature may be maintained over a given period of time; such "temperature programming" is frequently of value when complex mixtures of compounds having widely different volatilization characteristics are being examined. Columns of different lengths are commonly employed, varying from as little as 0.5 m to almost 3 m for packed and from 10 to 100 m for capillary columns; for many pharmaceutical applications a column of about 1.5 m is generally used and it may be from 2 to 5 mm in internal diameter.

The packing contained within columns for gas-liquid chromatography has a profound effect on the quality and effectiveness of separations. The solid support, which may vary in particle size from about 75 μm to 250 μm (60–200 mesh; although in any given column it should be closely defined within a narrow range), must be as inert as possible, particularly when polar drugs are to be chromatographed on supports coated with low concentrations of a liquid of low polarity. Active sites on the solid support may result in peak tailing of the solute, or even in its decomposition or rearrangement. Reactivity of the support may be minimized by treatment with a silanizing reagent before it is coated with the stationary phase. Injection residues might render the inlet part of the column ineffective.

Liquid phases commonly used include macrogols (polyethylene glycols) and esters, high molecular weight amides, silicone gums and fluids, and hydrocarbons. The silicone gums are substituted polysiloxanes and are a particularly valuable series of stationary phases. The highest temperature at which the stationary phase is designed to be used should be carefully noted and respected since "column bleeding" may occur and vitiate results if excessive temperatures are used. Prior to use a new column should be conditioned by maintaining it for several hours with a stream of carrier gas passing throught it at a temperature somewhat higher than the temperature at which the column is subsequently to be used but certainly not above the highest recommended temperature.

As carrier gas it is necessary to choose one that is inert and for flame-ionization detection (the most commonly used method in pharmaceutical analysis), nitrogen is very satisfactory. Though helium is also suitable and is actually to be preferred for work with a thermal conductivity detector because of its high thermal conductivity, it is expensive and not readily available in all parts of the world, whereas nitrogen is.

For quantitative applications of gas-liquid chromatography in the pharmacopoeia an internal standard is usually used since the comparison of one chromatogram with another resulting from a second injection on to the column could be subject to error. The addition of a suitable internal standard to the test solution and to a standard solution eliminates this error since the ratio of area or height (see below) of the peak due to the substance to be determined and of that due to the internal standard is compared from one chromatogram to another. In other applications it may be more convenient to use a process of normalization (particularly where an impurity is being assessed). In this case, the area of the peak due to the sought-for impurity is expressed as a percentage of the total area of all peaks derived from the substance being examined and its attendant impurities. Since the peak due to the principal component will usually be at least two orders of magnitude greater than that due to a minor impurity, it is necessary for such determinations to use a reliable automatic integrator and a wide-range amplifier that will respond in a linear fashion to both the major and the minor components. Peak areas may also be determined by planimeter, graphically, or by comparing the weights of paper cut from underneath the various peaks. In certain circumstances, it may be valid to use measurements of peak height rather than peak area, although the latter is considered to be more accurate for quantitative determinations. When the measurement of peak width is required, it is defined as the distance along the base line that is between the two points of intersection of lines drawn tangentially to the sides of the peak.

When the internal standard method is used the detailed procedure given below is applicable. It will be noted that reference is made to 3 solutions. The first of these (solution 1) contains an internal standard and an appropriate quantity of the substance to be determined (in the case of an impurity determination this might be the impurity itself, if available, or a suitably low loading of the substance in which impurities are to be sought). Chromatogram A thus obtained permits the relationship of response to the internal standard and to the substance being determined to be established. The second solution (solution 2) consists only of the substance being examined; this enables the analyst to confirm that there is no impurity present that will elute with the same retention time as the internal standard or to make allowance for the quantity present if there is a coincident peak. The third solution (solution 3) consists of the substance being examined and the internal standard (the latter present at the same concentration as in solution 1). Data derived from chromatograms A and C, corrected if necessary for observations made on chromatogram B, enable the quantities of minor constituents present in the substance being examined to be determined.

When a normalization procedure is used, a single solution may suffice since the total area of all minor peaks is to be expressed as a proportion of the total peak area. If a specific minor peak is to be evaluated, a second solution containing the sought-after material will be necessary so that the appropriate peak on the chromatogram of the substance being examined may be identified.

RECOMMENDED PROCEDURE

The length of the chromatographic column, the stationary phase, the solid support, the temperature, the carrier gas, the detector, and any other relevant details that are required for the determination are specified in the monograph. Where a non-volatile material is to be injected on to the column, a suitable interchangeable pre-column may be used.

In certain monographs a minimum column efficiency may be required. This is defined by the expression $16\ t_R^2/Ly^2$, where

t_R is the distance (in mm) along the base line between the point of injection and a perpendicular dropped from the maximum of the peak produced by the internal standard specified in the monograph;

L is the length (in m) of the column;

y is the peak width (in mm) of the peak produced by the internal standard.

When aqueous solutions are examined and a flame ionization detector is used, the results are invalid if the water is eluted at the same time as any of the required components.

Method

Using solution 1, determine experimentally suitable sensitivity settings of the instrument and the volumes of solutions to be injected to produce an adequate response. Adjustment of the concentration of the internal standard should be made, if necessary, so that the recorder response produced by the internal standard is approximately the same as the response of the susbtance being determined. Prepare a differential chromatogram by injecting the selected volume of solution 1 through the sample injection port on the chromatographic column, maintained at a suitable temperature, and eluting with the carrier gas. Repeat the determination twice more. In the same manner, prepare graphs using the same volumes of solutions 2 and 3. Measure the peak areas or, where the symmetry factor lies between 0.95 and 1.05, the peak heights produced by the substance or substances being determined and the internal standard. If an impurity peak has the same retention time as the internal standard, allowance is made in assessing the responses of these constituents for the contribution of each. From the values obtained calculate the proportion of the substance or substances being determined.

The symmetry factor of a peak is calculated from the expression $y_x/2A$, where:

y_x is the width of the peak at one-twentieth of the peak height;

A is the distance between the perpendicular dropped from the peak maximum and the leading edge of the peak at one-twentieth of the peak height.

The results of the determination are usually not valid unless the resolution between measured peaks on the chromatogram is greater than 1.0. The resolution is calculated from the expression $2(t_{Rb} - t_{Ra})/(Y_a + Y_b)$, where :

t_{Ra} and t_{Rb} are the distances along the base line between the point of injection and perpendiculars dropped from the maxima of two adjacent peaks;

Y_a and Y_b are the respective peak widths.

DETERMINATION OF pH

A value characteristic of an aqueous solution is its pH value, which represents conventionally its acidity or alkalinity.

The pH of a solution is the negative logarithm of the hydrogen ion activity, which may be measured potentiometrically. Formerly, pH was regarded as the negative logarithm of the hydrogen ion concentration. As it is known that not all hydrogen ions are necessarily equally active, this concentration may be different from the hydrogen ion activity. However, if the activity coefficient is close to 1, as is true in dilute solutions, the values of hydrogen ion activity and hydrogen ion concentration become nearly identical.

The determination of the pH value is carried out by measurement of the potential difference between electrodes immersed in standard and test solutions. The standard solutions used are assigned a definite pH value by convention.

In the measurement of pH, glass electrode finds wide applicability as it shows an immediate response to rapid changes of hydrogen ion concentrations even in poorly buffered solutions. Since the mechanism of this electrode involves no electron exchange it is the only electrode sensitive to hydrogen ions that is not disturbed by oxidizing or reducing agents.

The pH values of solutions or suspensions that are only partially aqueous and that can be considered only as "apparent pH values" can also be measured by using the proper electrode and by suitably standardizing the pH-meter.

As pH values are dependent on temperature, the measurements are carried out at selected constant temperatures.

Solutions used in determinations of pH are prepared with carbon-dioxide-free water R.

pH Scale

The difference in pH between two solutions, X and S, at the same temperature may be defined operationally as follows:

The electromotive force E_x, of the cell

Pt | H_2 | solution X | 3.5 mol/l KCl | reference electrode

and the electromotive force, E_s, of the cell

Pt | H_2 | solution S | 3.5 mol/l KCl | reference electrode

are measured, both cells being at the same temperature throughout and the reference electrodes and bridge solutions being identical in the two cells.

The pH of solution X, denoted by pH (X), is then related to the pH of solution S, denoted by pH (S), by the equation:

$$\text{pH}\,(X) = \text{pH}\,(S) + \frac{E_x - E_s}{2.3026\,RT/F}$$

where R denotes the gas constant, T the thermodynamic temperature (in K), and F the Faraday constant. Thus defined, the quantity pH is a dimensionless number.

Numerical values of the factor $2.3026\,RT/F$ at several temperatures are given below:

Temperature (in °C)	2.3026 RT/F (mV)
10	56.18
15	57.17
20	58.17
25	59.16
30	60.15

Potentiometric Determination of pH

For the practical determination of pH, a potentiometric method is usually employed. When glass electrodes are used they should be stored in a suitable liquid, usually water.

It is often found more convenient to measure pH by means of a glass electrode instead of the hydrogen electrode. In some solutions, especially those containing oxidizing agents, the glass electrode can be used when the hydrogen electrode cannot. The accuracy and reproducibility of $\pm$ 0.005 usually obtainable with the hydrogen electrode are, however, rarely obtainable with the glass electrode, and never outside the pH range 2–10.

When the glass electrode is used, the best accuracy is obtained by assuming that over a short range of pH there is a linear relation between pH and measured electromotive force, but that the proportionality factor relating them is not necessarily exactly 2.3026 RF/T. This method of using the glass electrode necessitates calibration by means of two solutions of known pH, near to, and preferably bracketing, the pH to be measured. There are at present various suitable solutions, the pH values of which are reliably known to an accuracy of $\pm$ 0.005 (see Table 3).

TABLE 3. STANDARD BUFFER SOLUTIONS AND THEIR pH VALUES

Standard buffer solutions	pH values at various temperatures				
	20 °C	25 °C	30 °C	35 °C	40 °C
Potassium tetraoxalate standard TS	1.675	1.679	1.683	1.688	1.694
Potassium hydrogen tartrate standard TS	—	3.557	3.552	3.549	3.547
Potassium hydrogen phthalate standard TS	4.002	4.008	4.015	4.024	4.035
Phosphate standard buffer, pH 6.8, TS	6.881	6.865	6.853	6.844	6.838
Phosphate standard buffer, pH 7.4, TS	7.429	7.413	7.400	7.389	7.380
Sodium tetraborate standard TS	9.225	9.180	9.139	9.102	9.068
Sodium carbonate standard TS	10.062	10.012	9.966	9.925	9.889

Calibration of apparatus

The apparatus is calibrated with standard buffer solutions to check the linearity of the response of the electrode at different pH values and to detect a faulty glass electrode. The standardization of the apparatus with only a single solution may be completely erroneous and therefore at least two standard buffer solutions should be used for calibration. The presence of a faulty electrode will be detected by failure to obtain a reasonably correct value ($\pm$ 0.04 unit) for the pH of the second standard solution when the apparatus has been standardized in terms of the first standard. A cracked electrode will yield pH values that are essentially the same for both solutions. If the difference between the known and the observed pH values for the second solution exceeds $\pm$ 0.04, another glass electrode should be substituted. If the difference persists, fresh standard solutions should be prepared.

RECOMMENDED PROCEDURE

After the apparatus has been calibrated, thoroughly wash the electrodes and the cup. Fill the cup with a portion of the solution to be tested and obtain a preliminary value for the pH. In general, this value will drift and is regarded as an approximation. Subsequent readings taken on additional portions of the same solution will yield successively more constant pH values. In the case of solutions that are well buffered, 3 portions may be sufficient to yield pH values that are reproducible to $\pm$ 0.04 unit and that show drifts of less than $\pm$ 0.04 unit in 1 or 2 minutes. In the case of very dilute or unbuffered solutions, as many as 6 portions of the test solution may be required, and the pH values may continue to drift and be reproducible to only $\pm$ 0.05 unit.

If a precision greater than 0.1 pH unit is desired, the temperature of the standard solutions, the glass and calomel electrodes, and the test solutions must be within 2 °C of one another, and the electrodes, standard solutions, test solutions, and wash water must be kept at the temperature of measurement for at least 2 hours prior to making the measurement in order to reduce to a negligible value the effects of thermal or electrical hysteresis of the electrodes.

Standard buffer solutions

Standard buffer solutions are used in the determination of pH values. They are prepared with carbon-dioxide-free water R. They should be stored in bottles of chemically resistant glass or in bottles made of polyethylene.

Unless otherwise specified, standard buffer solutions should not be used later than 3 months, after preparation. If growth of microorganisms starts in the solutions they should immediately be discarded and the bottles thoroughly cleaned and sterilized before refilling.

ELECTROPHORESIS

Electrophoresis is a physical method of analysis permitting the separation of compounds that are capable of acquiring en electrical charge in a conducting electrolyte. In this medium the ionized particles move more or less rapidly under the influence of an electrical field.

The electrophoretic mobility is the rate of migration of the substance measured in cm/s under the influence of a potential gradient of 1 V/cm, and is expressed in $cm^2 \cdot V^{-1} \cdot s^{-1}$.

The measurement of electrophoretic mobility is significant only where experimental conditions have been precisely defined. This mobility depends on the characteristics of the substance, its nature, size, form, and electrical charge. It also depends on the composition of the conducting liquid, its nature, concentration, pH, the presence of additional solvents and viscosity. The direction of migration depends on the sign of the electrical charge of the particle as it moves towards the electrode of opposite sign.

According to the methods used, the electrophoretic mobility is either measured directly or compared with that of a reference substance.

Moving Boundary (Free-flow) Electrophoresis

This technique, used exclusively for the determination of the mobility, is particularly suitable for substances of high molecular weight with poor diffusion properties.

The boundaries are usually measured both before and after the application of an electrical field by a physical method, such as refractometry or conductometry. The concentration of the substance in the conducting liquid, the characteristics of the latter and the details of the procedure, including quantitative evaluation of the fractions, are specified in the monographs.

Zone Electrophoresis (Electrophoresis using a Supporting Medium)

This method uses only small sample sizes. The nature of the supporting medium (for example, paper, cellulose acetate, starch-gel, agar-gel, polymethacrylamide, mixed gel) introduces additional factors influencing the mobility. The rate of migration depends on the mobility of the particles and also on the electro-endosmotic current (in the case of carriers with polar properties), on the currents due to evaporation (caused by heat generated through the Joule effect), and on the gradient of the electrical field.

In practice, the mobility of the electrophoretic zones and their signs are ignored; the zones are located by experience or by comparison with those given by a reference substance treated in the same way.

After separation of the constituents the position of colourless substances may be determined by treating the electropherogram with a reagent that will convert them to coloured or fluorescent derivatives. For quantitative purposes, the spot (zone) may be carefully separated, the substance eluted with a suitable solvent and then determined by a sufficiently sensitive method, such as spectrophotometric measurement, either directly or after a chemical reaction. In another quantitative procedure after conversion to a coloured derivative, the zone intensity can be measured with the aid of a scanning densitometer.

An apparatus for electrophoresis on a supporting medium is composed of:

• A source of direct current, preferably of stabilized voltage.

• A chamber for electrophoresis, generally in the form of a parallel-epiped, made from glass or rigid plastic material with an airtight lid ensuring the maintenance of an atmosphere of saturated humidity. Two insulated electrical leads are sealed through the walls of the chamber, one at either end, each lead having an internal connector to which are attached electrodes of platinum wire. The chamber should be fitted with suitable safety devices to ensure that the electrical supply is discon-nected when the lid is removed. Two double troughs provided with a central lengthwise partition are inserted in the chamber, one at each end. Alternatively, the troughs may be integral parts of the chamber. One platinum electrode is laid along the bottom of each outer trough compartment. The electrodes are connected through external insulated cables to an electrical power source having an output of not less than 450 V D.C. at 150 mA. The power source should be provided with a means of indicating and controlling the voltage and of indicating the current consumption. Additional circuitry may be incorporated to stabilize the voltage.

• A holder device. When paper or cellulose acetate is used, the carrier strips impregnated with the conducting liquid are stretched by an appropriate arrangement and the ends immersed into the electrode troughs. In gel electrophoresis, an adherent on an even layer of gel is placed on glass and the electrical connexions are attached at each end.

• A device to locate and measure the spots.

RECOMMENDED PROCEDURES

Paper electrophoresis

A chamber about 50 cm long, 38 cm wide and 4.5 cm deep, with troughs about 37 cm long externally, 5 cm wide and 2 cm in depth intern-ally, is suitable.

The electrophoresis paper consists of suitable filter-paper (Whatman 3 MM or similar grade is suitable) that has been washed chromatographically with a suitable solvent if so specified in the monograph. The paper is cut into strips of appropriate size and a base line is drawn across the paper about 13 cm from one end.

Fill the troughs of the apparatus with the conducting liquid specified in the monograph. Place strips of electrophoresis paper (about 30 cm by 5 cm) in the troughs so as to form bridges between the outer and inner compartments and ensure that the electrodes are fully immersed in the conducting liquid in the outer compartments.

Apply separately to points along the base line of the electrophoresis paper, at least 1 cm from the edge of the paper and not less than 2.5 cm apart, the volumes of solutions prepared as specified in the monograph.

Allow the spots to dry and then place the end of the paper nearest the base line in the inner compartment of the trough connected to the anode and the other end in the inner compartment of the trough connected to the cathode. Wet the paper with the conducting liquid, using a brush, starting from the ends of the paper and working towards the base line. Do not wet the strip that includes the applied substance. Close the lid, allow the liquid to diffuse across the base line, if necessary cover the apparatus so as to exclude light, connect the cables to the power supply and switch on the current. Adjust the voltage to about 20 V per cm of paper between the troughs and allow electrophoresis to proceed for the time indicated or until the marker substances have moved the specified distances. Switch off the current, remove the paper, dry in a current of air protected from light if necessary, and examine the resulting electropherogram under the conditions prescribed in the monograph. When the use of marker substances is specified, the test is valid only if the marker substances move to the specified distances from the base line. If the intensity of any subsidiary spots derived from the tested substance is less than that of the spot obtained from the reference solution, the substance conforms to the requirements. When specified in the monograph, spray the paper uniformly on both sides with the reagent, carry out any further prescribed treatment to complete the reaction, and apply the same criteria to the resulting spots.

Electrophoresis on cellulose acetate strips

It is preferable to use a smaller chamber than for paper electrophoresis; one measuring about 25 cm by 24 cm with troughs of 10 cm by 23 cm is suitable.

Use cellulose polyacetate strips of suitable quality, measuring 2.5 cm by 17 cm, which are immersed in the conducting liquid for approximately 1 hour before use.

Apply the solutions, prepared as specified in the monograph and in the volume indicated, 8 cm from one end of the strip, then carry out electrophoresis as described under paper electrophoresis. Colour the bands, wash them and render them transparent by the methods specified in the monographs, which also give the method of evaluation to be used.

Gel electrophoresis

The inert carrier consists of a 1–2 mm thick layer of an agar or starch gel of suitable consistency and shaped as an elongated rectangle.

The conducting liquid is either incorporated into the gel layer or sprinkled on it, until it is well moistened, after it has already been formed. The solution of the substance is placed on the surface of the gel layer or inside the holes bored for that purpose in the layer. The gel layer is connected at both its narrower ends with two troughs containing the conducting liquid, the connexion being made by wicks composed of a double layer of absorbent lint moistened with the conducting liquid. The gel layer on its support and the connexions are then placed in a suitable chamber.

The electrophoretic process is effected by application of direct electric current. To remove heat generated by the Joule effect of the current, water or other suitable cooling liquid should be circulated in the course of the process through the supporting plate.

When the process has been completed, the resulting spots or areas of migration are located by a suitable method (for example, as an inhibition zone after suitable incubation, if the tested substance is an antibiotic and an appropriate test organism has been incorporated into the gel layer, or by a chemical method), as specified in the individual monographs.

PHASE SOLUBILITY ANALYSIS

Phase solubility analysis is a technique for quantitatively determining the purity of a substance through the application of precise solubility measurements. At a given temperature, a definite amount of a pure substance is soluble in a definite quantity of solvent. The resulting solution is saturated in respect of the particular substance, but the solution remains unsaturated in respect of other substances even though such substances may be closely related in chemical structure and physical properties to the particular substance being tested. Constancy of solubility indicates that a material is pure or free from foreign substances except in the unique case where the percentage composition of the material being tested is in direct ratio to the solubilities of the respective components. Conversely, variability of solubility indicates the presence of an impurity or impurities.

The standard solubility method consists of several distinct steps: (*a*) preparation of a series of separate systems composed of increasing quantities of material and measured, constant amounts of solvent; (*b*) establishment of equilibrium for each system at identical constant temperature and pressure; (*c*) separation of the solid phase from the solutions; (*d*) determination of the concentration of the material dissolved in the various solutions; (*e*) graphical representation of the ratio of the weight of the dissolved materials per weight of solvent against the ratio of the total weight of material per weight of solvent, extrapolation and calculation. Alternatively, statistical procedures may be used to evaluate the purity of the test substance from the data obtained.

Solvents

The following criteria are used in the selection of a proper solvent for phase solubility analysis:

(1) The solvent should be of such volatility that it can be evaporated under vacuum, but it should not be so volatile that difficulty is experienced in transferring and weighing the solvent and its solutions. Normally, solvents with boiling points between 60 °C and 150 °C are suitable.

(2) The solvent should not adversely affect the substance. Solvents that cause decomposition or react with the substance cannot be used. Solvents that solvate or form salts should be avoided if possible.

(3) The solvent should be of known purity and composition. Mixed solvents are permissible. Trace impurities may affect solubility greatly.

(4) For the method described below the test substance should be soluble to the extent of not less than 4 mg/g and not more than 50 mg/g in the solvent chosen. A solubility of 10–20 mg/g is optimal.

Apparatus

Constant-temperature bath. For these tests use a constant-temperature bath capable of maintaining a preselected temperature within ± 0.1 °C. Normally temperatures of 25 °C or 30 °C are selected. The bath should be equipped with a horizontal shaft capable of rotating at approximately 25 revolutions per minute, equipped with clamps to hold ampoules. Alternatively the bath may contain a suitable vibrator, capable of vibrating at 100–120 vibrations per second, equipped with a shaft with suitable clamps to hold the ampoules, or other suitable device to achieve equilibrium in the ampoules.

Ampoules. Use 15-ml ampoules similar to that shown in Fig. 2. Other containers may be used provided that they are leakproof and are suitable in all other respects.

FIG. 2. AMPOULE (LEFT) AND SOLUBILITY FLASK (RIGHT)
USED IN PHASE SOLUBILITY ANALYSIS

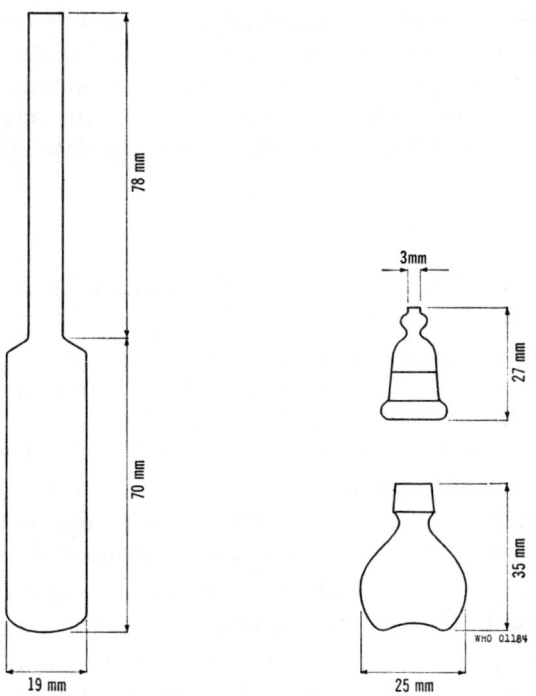

Solubility flasks. Use solubility flasks suitable for freeze-drying. A suitable flask (with stopper) is shown in Fig. 2.

Balance. Use a suitable balance and technique to ensure that all weighings are within ± 10 μg.

RECOMMENDED PROCEDURE

The method described below is generally applicable. However, in certain cases other conditions (volume of solvent, etc.) than those specified here might be preferable.

System composition

Weigh accurately not less than 7 marked, scrupulously cleaned, ampoules and into each of them weigh, accurately, increasingly larger amounts of the test substance. The weight of the test substance is selected so that the first ampoule contains slightly less material than will go into solution in 5 ml of the selected solvent, and the second ampoule and subsequent ampoules slightly more than the indicated solubility. Pipette 5.0 ml of the solvent into each of the ampoules, cool in a dry-ice/acetone mixture, and seal, using a double-jet air-gas burner and taking care to save all the fragments of glass. Allow the ampoules and their contents to come to room temperature, and weigh the individual sealed ampoules plus any corresponding glass fragments. Calculate the system composition, in mg of substance per g of solvent, for each ampoule by the formula $1000\ (W_2 - W_1)/(W_3 - W_2)$, in which W_1 is the weight of the empty ampoule, W_2 is the weight of the ampoule plus test substance, and W_3 is the weight of the ampoule plus test substance, solvent and separated glass.

Equilibration

The time required for equilibration varies with the substance, the method of mixing (vibration or rotation) and the temperature. Normally equilibrium is obtained more rapidly by the vibration method (1–7 days) than by the rotational method (7–14 days).

In order to demonstrate that a state of equilibrium has been attained, the following procedure is frequently applicable: Bring about a super-saturated solution in one of the ampoules — the next to the last in the series — by warming it to a temperature about 10 °C above that of the constant-temperature bath, taking care that not all the solid in the ampoule is dissolved. Thereafter, treat this ampoule in exactly the same manner as the other ampoules. If the solubility value obtained from it plots out in line with the other values, it indicates that all the ampoules have attained equilibrium. However, failure of the solubility value from the "supersaturated" ampoule to fall in line with the other solubility values does not necessarily prove that the other ampoules have not attained equilibrium, since it can occasionally be due to the tendency of certain materials to remain in supersaturated solution. To attain equilibrium in such cases, run a series of phase solubility analyses applying different equilibration times so as to make certain that constant values for the slope of the solubility curve have been achieved.

Solution composition

After equilibration, place the ampoules vertically in a rack in the constant-temperature bath, with their necks above the water level, and allow the contents to settle. Taking full precautions to minimize solvent evaporation, open the ampoules, and remove a volume of 2.0 ml from each by means of a pipette equipped with a small pledget of cotton-wool or with other suitable means of serving as a filter. Remove the cotton-wool, transfer the aliquot of clear solution from each ampoule to a marked, tared solubility flask, and weigh each flask plus its solution to obtain the weight of the solution. Cool the flasks in a dry-ice/acetone bath, and then evaporate the solvent in a vacuum. Gradually increase the temperature from 70 to 100 °C, and dry the residue to constant weight. Calculate the solution composition, in mg of substance per g of solvent, by the formula $1000 (F_3 - F_1)/(F_2 - F_3)$, in which F_1 is the weight of the solubility flask, F_2 is the weight of the flask plus solution, and F_3 is the weight of the flask plus residue.

Calculation

Prepare a graphical representation of the results for each portion of the test substance taken by plotting the ratio of the weight of the dissolved materials per weight of solvent (Y axis or solution composition) against the ratio of the total weight of material per weight of solvent (X axis or system composition). As shown in Fig. 3, the points for those containers that represent a true solution should approach a straight line (AB) with a

FIG. 3. TYPICAL PHASE SOLUBILITY DIAGRAM

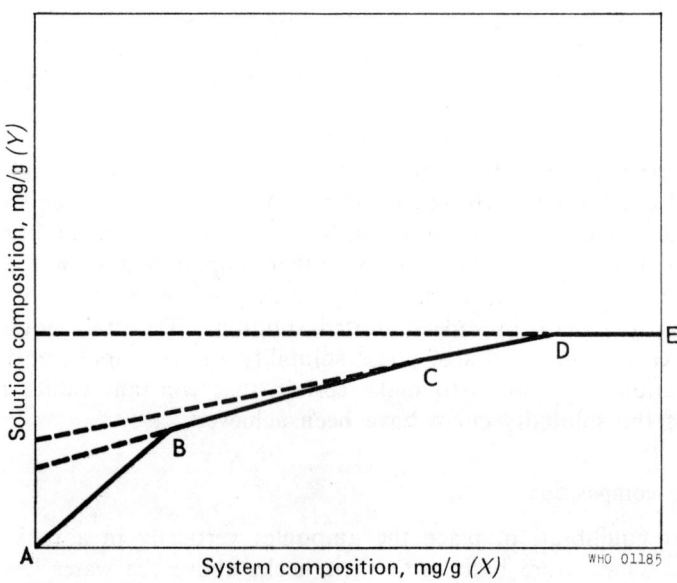

slope of 1, passing through the origin; the points corresponding to saturated solutions should approach another straight line (BC), the slope, S, of which represents the fraction of total impurities present in the test substance. Failure of points to approach a straight line usually indicates that equilibrium has not been achieved although this may also be due to formation of a solid solution or departure from ideal behaviour. Calculate the percentage purity of the test substance by the formula $100-100S$. The slope may be calculated by the equation $S = (Y_2 - Y_1)/(X_2 - X_1)$ in which Y_2 and Y_1 represent solution compositions, and X_2 and X_1 represent the respective system compositions, at convenient points on the second straight line (BC).

The point B in the diagram represents the system where the main component or, in rare cases, the least soluble of the components of the test substance has reached the limit of its solubility. The solubility of this component is obtained by extending the solubility line (BC) through the Y axis. The point of interception on the Y axis gives the solubility, in mg/g, which should be constant for a given compound.

At point C in the diagram the next component of the test substance has reached the limit of its solubility. The intercept obtained by extending the solubility line (CD) through the Y axis represents the combined solubilities of the two components that have first reached their solubility limits. The solubility of the second component can thus be obtained by subtraction.

Between points D and E in the diagram the solution is saturated in respect of all components in the test substance, and its composition remains constant.

Under appropriate conditions the number of impurities present in the test substance is shown by the number of inflexions of the solubility curve above the first saturation point (B) and the solubilities of the respective components can be obtained in a way similar to that described above.

CHEMICAL METHODS

GENERAL IDENTIFICATION TESTS

Acetylated substances

Place a quantity of the substance as specified in the monograph in a test-tube (of maximum 18 mm diameter) and treat it with 3 drops of phosphoric acid ($\sim$1440 g/l) TS. Close the tube with a stopper through which passes a smaller test-tube filled with water and on the outside of which hangs a drop of lanthanum nitrate (30 g/l) TS. Heat the apparatus in a boiling water-bath for 5 minutes. Transfer the drop of lanthanum nitrate to a white porcelain spot plate and mix with a drop of iodine (0.02 mol/l) VS. Place at the edge of the mixture a drop of ammonia ($\sim$100 g/l) TS. A blue colour slowly appears at the interface of the two liquids and persists for a short time.

Amines, primary aromatic

Dissolve a quantity of the substance as specified in the monograph in 2 ml of hydrochloric acid ($\sim$70 g/l) TS with the aid of heat, if necessary. Cool in ice, treat it with 4 ml of sodium nitrite (10 g/l) TS and pour the mixture into 2 ml of 2-naphthol TS1 containing 1 g of sodium acetate R. A heavy precipitate, coloured as specified in the monograph, is produced.

Ammonia and volatile aliphatic amines

Dissolve a quantity of the substance as specified in the monograph, place the solution in a test-tube and add 1 g of magnesium oxide R; warm, if specified in the monograph. Alkaline vapours evolve gradually and turn manganese/silver paper R black, the reagent paper being placed in the upper part of the test-tube.

Ammonium

Carry out the test in an apparatus consisting of stoppered test-tubes A and B connected by a bent glass tube to permit a stream of air to pass consecutively through test-tubes A and B.

Place the solution as specified in the monograph and 0.2 g of magnesium oxide R into test-tube A, and 1 ml of hydrochloric acid (0.1 mol/l) VS containing 1 drop of methyl red/ethanol TS in test-tube B. Bubble air through the apparatus. Evolved ammonia turns the colour of the solution in test-tube B to yellow. On the addition of 1 ml of sodium cobaltinitrite (100 g/l) TS to this solution a yellowish brown precipitate is formed.

Bismuth

A. Prepare the solution in hydrochloric acid (∼250 g/l) TS as specified in the monograph and dilute 10 times with water. A white precipitate is formed, which turns dark brown on the addition of sodium sulfide TS.

B. Treat the solution in nitric acid (∼1000 g/l) TS as specified in the monograph with potassium iodide (80 g/l) TS. A black precipitate is formed, which is soluble in an excess of the reagent to give a yellowish brown or orange solution. Dilute this solution with several volumes of water and heat; an orange or copper-coloured precipitate is obtained. The black precipitate that is first formed on the addition of potassium iodide (80 g/l) TS also becomes orange or copper-coloured when heated with water.

Bromides

A. Prepare a solution as specified in the monograph, acidify with nitric acid (∼130 g/l) TS and add silver nitrate (40 g/l) TS. A yellowish curdy precipitate is produced, which is partially soluble in ammonia (∼260 g/l) TS, but almost insoluble in ammonia (∼100 g/l) TS and in nitric acid (∼1000 g/l) TS.

B. (For testing bromides or hydrobromides of insoluble or sparingly soluble bases). Prepare the solution as specified in the monograph, add ammonia (∼100 g/l) TS, filter, acidify the filtrate with nitric acid (∼130 g/l) TS, and proceed with test A.

C. Prepare the solution as specified in the monograph, acidify with sulfuric acid (∼100 g/l)TS, and mix with chlorine TS. A brown solution results; after shaking with chloroform R it becomes colourless, whereas the chloroform layer turns reddish.

Calcium

A. Prepare the solution as specified in the monograph and add to it ammonium oxalate (25 g/l) TS. A white precipitate is formed, which is soluble in hydrochloric acid (∼250 g/l) TS but is practically insoluble in acetic acid (∼300 g/l) TS.

B. Treat 1 drop of a solution as specified in the monograph with 4 drops of glyoxal bis(2-hydroxyanil) TS, and 1 drop of sodium hydroxide (∼80 g/l)TS. A reddish brown precipitate is formed, which dissolves in chloroform R to give a red solution.

Chlorides

A. Prepare a solution as specified in the monograph, acidify with nitric acid (∼130 g/l) TS and add silver nitrate (40 g/l) TS. A white curdy precipitate is produced, which is soluble in ammonia (~100 g/l) TS but is practically insoluble in nitric acid (~1000 g/l) TS.

B. (For testing chlorides or hydrochlorides of insoluble or sparingly soluble bases). Prepare the solution as specified in the monograph, add ammonia (~100 g/l) TS, filter and acidify the filtrate with nitric acid (~130 g/l) TS and proceed with test A.

C. Mix the quantity of the substance as specified in the monograph with an equal quantity of manganese dioxide R, moisten with sulfuric acid (~1760 g/l) TS and heat gently. The evolved chlorine is recognizable by its greenish colour and produces a blue coloration of moistened starch/iodide paper R. Carry out the reaction preferably under a hood.

Citrates

A. Treat at ambient temperature a neutral solution as specified in the monograph with calcium chloride (55 g/l) TS. No precipitate is formed, but on boiling, a white solid is produced, which is soluble in acetic acid (~300 g/l) TS.

B. Boil a solution with mercuric sulfate TS as specified in the monograph and filter if necessary. After the addition of a few drops of potassium permanganate (10 g/l) TS to the filtrate, the colour is discharged and a white precipitate is produced.

Ferrous salts

A. Prepare a solution as specified in the monograph and add potassium ferricyanide (10 g/l) TS. A dark-blue precipitate is formed, which is practically insoluble in hydrochloric acid (~70 g/l)TS.

B. Prepare a solution as specified in the monograph, acidify with sulfuric acid (~100 g/l) TS, and treat with o-phenanthroline (1 g/l) TS. An intense red colour is produced, which is discharged by the addition of ceric sulfate (35 g/l) TS.

Iodides

A. Prepare a solution as specified in the monograph, acidify with nitric acid (~130 g/l) TS and add silver nitrate (40 g/l) TS. A yellow curdy precipitate is formed, which is practically insoluble in ammonia (~100 g/l) TS and in nitric acid (~1000 g/l) TS.

B. (For testing iodides of insoluble or sparingly soluble bases). Prepare the solution as specified in the monograph, add ammonia (~100 g/l) TS, filter and acidify the filtrate with nitric acid (~130 g/l) TS and proceed with test A.

C. Prepare a solution as specified in the monograph, acidify with sulfuric acid ($\sim$100 g/l) TS and add potassium nitrite (100 g/l) TS. A brown solution results; after shaking with chloroform R, it becomes colourless, whereas the chloroform layer turns violet.

Nitrates

A. Prepare a solution as specified in the monograph and treat it with ferrous sulfate (15 g/l) TS. No brown colour appears unless sulfuric acid ($\sim$1760 g/l) TS is cautiously added to form a lower layer. A brown colour is then produced at the interface of the two liquids.

B. Add 2 mg of the finely ground test substance to a mixture of 0.1 ml of nitrobenzene R and 0.2 ml of sulfuric acid ($\sim$ 1760 g/l) TS. Allow to stand at room temperature for 5 minutes, cool in ice, and add slowly while mixing 5 ml of water and 3 ml of sodium hydroxide ($\sim$400 g/l) TS. Add 5 ml of acetone R, shake and allow to separate. An intense violet colour is produced in the upper phase.

Orthophosphates

A. Add drop by drop a quantity of nitric acid ($\sim$130 g/l) TS to 5 ml of ammonium molybdate (95 g/l) TS until any precipitate that may appear dissolves. Divide this solution into 2 portions, add to one portion the test solution acidified with nitric acid ($\sim$130 g/l) TS as specified in the monograph, and boil both portions. A yellow precipitate is formed with the test solution while the other shows no more than a slight opalescence.

B. Prepare a neutral solution as specified in the monograph and add silver nitrate (40 g/l) TS. A yellow precipitate is produced, which does not darken upon heating the solution to boiling. The precipitate is soluble in ammonia ($\sim$100 g/l) TS and in nitric acid ($\sim$130 g/l) TS.

Potassium

Prepare an alkaline solution as specified in the monograph and treat it with sodium tetraphenylborate (30 g/l) TS. A white precipitate is produced.

Salicylates

Treat a neutral solution as specified in the monograph with ferric chloride (25 g/l) TS. An intense reddish violet colour appears, which remains on the addition of a small amount of acetic acid ($\sim$300 g/l) TS but disappears on the addition of hydrochloric acid ($\sim$70 g/l) TS, with separation of a white crystalline precipitate.

Sodium

A. Moisten a quantity of the substance with hydrochloric acid ($\sim$250 g/l) TS. An intense yellow colour is produced when the solution is introduced into a nonluminous flame.

NOTE : Perform test B if for technical reasons test A cannot be carried out.

B. Acidify a solution as specified in the monograph with acetic acid ($\sim$60 g/l) TS, filter, if necessary, and treat it with uranyl/zinc acetate TS. A yellow crystalline precipitate is produced.

Sulfates

A. Prepare a solution as specified in the monograph and add barium chloride (50 g/l) TS. A white precipitate is formed, which is practically insoluble in hydrochloric acid ($\sim$250 g/l) TS.

B. To a solution as specified in the monograph, add lead acetate (80 g/l) TS. A white precipitate is formed, which is soluble in ammonium acetate (80 g/l) TS and in sodium hydroxide ($\sim$80 g/l) TS, but practically insoluble in hot water.

Tartrates

A. Acidify a solution as specified in the monograph with acetic acid ($\sim$300 g/l) TS and add 1 drop of ferrous sulfate (15 g/l) TS, a few drops of hydrogen peroxide ($\sim$60 g/l) TS, and enough sodium hydroxide ($\sim$80 g/l) TS to make the solution alkaline. A purple or violet colour is produced.

B. Mix a few ml of sulfuric acid ($\sim$1760 g/l) TS with a few drops of resorcinol (20 g/l) TS and a few drops of potassium bromide (100 g/l) TS and add 2 or 3 drops of a solution as specified in the monograph. Warm the liquid in a water-bath for 5 to 10 minutes. An intense blue colour is produced. Cool the liquid and pour it into water. The solution becomes red.

LIMIT TEST FOR CHLORIDES

The limit test for chlorides is provided to demonstrate that the content of chlorides does not exceed the limit given in the individual monograph in terms of micrograms of chloride ions per gram of the substance being tested. The standard solution against which the comparison of opalescence is made contains 250 μg of Cl^-.

Carry out the test in matched flat-bottomed comparison tubes of transparent glass of about 70 ml capacity and about 23 mm internal diameter bearing a 45-ml and a 50-ml mark. Nessler cylinders complying with the above dimensions are suitable. The expression "matched tubes" means tubes that are matched as closely as possible in internal diameter and in all other respects.

Prepare a solution as specified in the monograph, transfer to a comparison tube, dilute to 50 ml with water and add 1 ml of silver nitrate (40 g/l) TS. Stir immediately with a glass rod, and set aside for 5 minutes, protected from direct sunlight. The opalescence produced is not greater than the similarly prepared standard opalescence when viewed down the vertical axis of the tube in diffused light against a black background.

Standard opalescence

Measure 5.0 ml of hydrochloric acid ClTS and 10 ml of nitric acid (~130 g/l) TS into a comparison tube. Dilute to 50 ml with water, and add 1 ml of silver nitrate (40 g/l) TS. Stir immediately with a glass rod and set aside for 5 minutes, protected from direct sunlight.

LIMIT TEST FOR SULFATES

The limit test for sulfates is provided to demonstrate that the content of sulfates does not exceed the limit given in the individual monograph in terms of micrograms of sulfates per gram of the substance being tested.

The solution against which the comparison of turbidity is made contains 480 μg of SO_4^{--} more than the standard barium sulfate suspension.

Carry out the test in matched flat-bottomed comparison tubes of transparent glass of about 70 ml capacity and about 23 mm internal diameter bearing a 45-ml and a 50-ml mark. Nessler cylinders complying with the above dimensions are suitable. The expression "matched tubes" means tubes that are matched as closely as possible in internal diameter and in all other respects.

Prepare a solution as specified in the monograph, transfer to a comparison tube, dilute to 45 ml with water and add 5 ml of barium sulfate suspension TS. Stir immediately with a glass rod, and set aside for 10 minutes.

The turbidity produced is not greater than the similarly prepared standard turbidity when viewed down the vertical axis of the tube in diffused light against a black background.

Standard turbidity

Measure 1.00 ml of sulfuric acid (0.005 mol/l) VS and 3 ml of hydrochloric acid (~70 g/l) TS into a comparison tube. Dilute to 45 ml with water, and add 5 ml of barium sulfate suspension TS. Stir immediately with a glass rod and set aside for 10 minutes.

LIMIT TEST FOR HEAVY METALS

The limit test for heavy metals is provided to demonstrate that the content of metallic impurities that are coloured by hydrogen sulfide does not exceed the heavy metals limit given in the individual monograph in terms of micrograms of lead per gram of the test substance.

The test consists of two consecutive operations: preparation of the test solution, and the colour development by reaction with hydrogen sulfide, followed by comparison of the colour obtained with that produced with standard lead solution.

The preparation of the test solution is carried out, as specified in the monograph, according to procedures 1 to 4 described below. A blank is prepared in a similar manner.

The reaction with hydrogen sulfide is carried out by mixing the test solution with freshly prepared hydrogen sulfide TS. The comparison of the colour thus obtained is carried out either by directly comparing the coloration of the liquid in suitable comparison tubes (Method A) or by comparing the intensity of coloration of spots obtained by filtering the liquid using an appropriate apparatus (Method B).

Method A is generally applicable only when the amount of heavy metals in the weight of test substance used exceeds 5 µg; for amounts of 2–5 µg of heavy metals Method B should be used.

The standard lead solution used in the test; dilute lead PbTS contains 10 µg of lead in 1 ml. When 0.1 ml of this solution is employed to prepare the standard for comparison with a solution of 1 g of the substance being tested, the standard solution thus prepared contains 1 µg of Pb and represents the equivalent of 1 µg of lead per g of the substance tested.

Apparatus

For determination of heavy metals by Method A carry out the test in matched flat-bottomed comparison tubes of transparent glass of about

70 ml capacity and about 23 mm internal diameter bearing a 40-ml and a 50-ml mark. Nessler cylinders complying with the above dimensions are suitable. The expression "matched tubes" means tubes that are matched as closely as possible in internal diameter and in all other respects. For mixing the solution use a stirring rod preferably having a loop at the lower end.

For determination of heavy metals by Method B use a 50-ml syringe made of suitable material (usually plastic) with a detachable plunger and a male Luer conical joint of 9 mm internal diameter at the lower end (Millipore syringe XX 11 050 05 is suitable) to which an adapter for filtration is attached.

The adapter is made of suitable material (a filtration adapter Millipore SX00 013 00 in polypropylene is suitable) and has a female joint for connecting it with the syringe. It is devised so as to be separable into two parts to permit the exchange of filters, the lower part containing a support for membrane filters 13 mm in diameter. A suitable prefilter (Millipore prefilter AP 2001 300 is suitable) and a membrane filter made of mixed cellulose esters, 13 mm in diameter, with a pore opening of 3 μm (a Millipore filter SSWP 013 00 is suitable) are used for the filtration.

RECOMMENDED PROCEDURES

Preparation of test solution

Procedure 1. Weigh the quantity of substance specified in the monograph, dissolve it in 25 ml of water, adjust the pH of the solution to 3–4 with acetic acid (~60 g/l) PbTS, or with ammonia (~100 g/l) PbTS, as necessary, then dilute to 40 ml with water and mix.

Procedure 2. Weigh the quantity of substance specified in the monograph, dissolve it in about 30 ml of solvent specified (ethanol (~750 g/l) TS, methanol R, acetone R, or dioxan R may be used), add 0.5 ml of acetic acid (~300 g/l) TS, and dilute to 40 ml with the solvent.

Procedure 3. Place the quantity of the substance specified in the monograph in a suitable crucible, preferably made of silica, and carefully ignite at a low temperature until the contents are thoroughly charred. The crucible may be loosely covered with a lid during the charring. Add to the contents of the crucible 2 ml of nitric acid (~1000 g/l) TS and 5 drops of sulfuric acid (~1760 g/l TS), and cautiously heat until white fumes are evolved, and then ignite, preferably in a muffle furnace, at 500 °C until all the carbon is burned off. Cool, add 2 ml of hydrochloric acid (~250 g/l) TS, and slowly evaporate in a water-bath to dryness. Moisten the residue with 1 drop of hydrochloric acid (~250 g/l) TS, add 10 ml of hot water, and digest for 2 minutes. Add, drop by drop, ammonia ($\sim$100 g/l) PbTS, until the pH of the solution is between 8 and 8.5, then add, drop by drop, acetic acid ($\sim$60 g/l) PbTS, to adjust the pH to between 3 and 4. Filter if necessary, wash the crucible and the filter with about 10 ml of water, dilute with water to 40 ml, and mix.

Procedure 4. Place the quantity of substance specified in the monograph in a suitable crucible, preferably made of silica, mix it well with about 0.5 g of magnesium oxide R and incinerate until a homogeneous white mass is obtained. If after 15 minutes of incineration the residue is still coloured, let the crucible cool, mix the contents well with a glass rod and resume heating. Next, dissolve the residue in hydrochloric acid ($\sim$70 g/l) TS, add, drop by drop, a solution of ammonia ($\sim$100 g/l) PbTS, until the pH of the solution is between 8 and 8.5, then add, also drop by drop, acetic acid ($\sim$60 g/l) PbTS, to adjust the pH to 3–4, filter, dilute with water to 40 ml, and mix.

Colour development and measurement

Method A

To 40 ml of the liquid contained in the comparison tube add 10 ml of freshly prepared hydrogen sulfide TS, mix and allow to stand for 5 minutes.

In another comparison tube place a volume of solution of dilute lead PbTS, containing the lead equivalent of the heavy metals limit specified in the monograph, dilute with water, adjust the pH with ammonia ($\sim$100 g/l) PbTS and acetic acid ($\sim$60 g/l) PbTS to 3–4; dilute with water or the solvent used to 40 ml, mix, add 10 ml of freshly prepared hydrogen sulfide TS, mix and allow to stand for 5 minutes.

Compare the colours by viewing down the vertical axis of the tube in diffused light against a white background, or by another suitable method. The colour of the test solution is not darker than that of the lead standard.

Method B

Take the filtration syringe, arrange the prefilter and the membrane filter as indicated in the diagram for prefiltration, remove the plunger from the syringe, place the test solution inside the syringe, replace the plunger, and filter the test solution slowly by exerting a regular pressure on the plunger. Collect the filtrate in a beaker or a test-tube. Open the adapter and check whether the membrane filter is free from impurities. If not, replace it and repeat the operation in the same manner. Then rearrange the prefilter and membrane filter as indicated in Fig. 4. Adjust the pH of the filtrate with ammonia ($\sim$100 g/l) PbTS and acetic acid ($\sim$60 g/l) PbTS to 3–4, add 10 ml of freshly prepared hydrogen sulfide TS, all the reagents previously filtered through a membrane filter, mix, allow to stand for 5 minutes, take out the plunger, place the solution inside the syringe, and filter it through the membrane filter by exerting slowly a regular and moderate pressure on the plunger. Open the adapter and take out the membrane filter.

FIG. 4. LIMIT TEST FOR HEAVY METALS: METHOD B

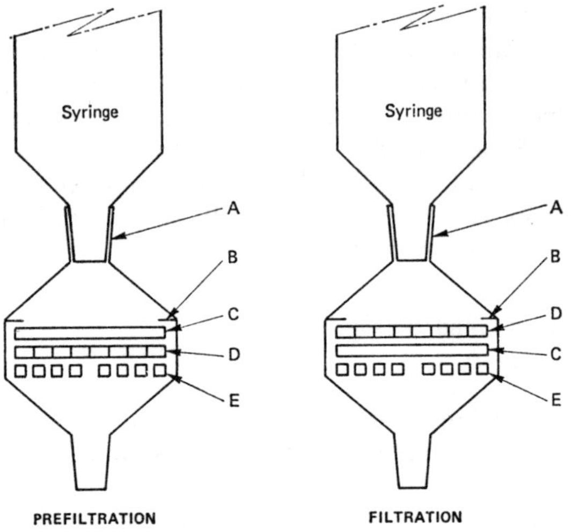

PREFILTRATION   FILTRATION

A — Luer cone
B — Joint
C — Prefilter
D — Membrane filter
E — Support

WHO 79050

Take a volume of solution of dilute lead PbTS containing the lead equivalent to the heavy metals limit specified in the monograph, dilute with water, adjust the pH with ammonia (∼100 g/l) PbTS and acetic acid (∼60 g/l) PbTS to 3–4, dilute with water to 40 ml, mix, and proceed as described above.

Compare the intensity of the coloration of spots obtained on the membrane filters. The colour obtained from the test solution is not more intense than that from the lead standard.

LIMIT TEST FOR IRON

The limit test for iron is provided to demonstrate that the content of iron does not exceed the limit given in the individual monograph in terms of micrograms of iron per gram of the test substance.

The standard solution against which the comparison of colour is made contains 40 µg of iron.

RECOMMENDED PROCEDURE

Carry out the test in matched flat-bottomed comparison tubes of transparent glass of about 70 ml capacity and about 23 mm internal diameter bearing a 45-ml and a 50-ml mark. Nessler cylinders complying with the above dimensions are suitable. The expression "matched tubes" means tubes that are matched as closely as possible in internal diameter and in all other respects.

Prepare the substance as specified in the monograph, or dissolve directly an indicated quantity in 40 ml of water, and transfer to a comparison tube. Add 2 ml of citric acid (180 g/l) FeTS and 2 drops of mercaptoacetic acid R; mix, make alkaline with ammonia (~100 g/l) FeTS, dilute to 50 ml with water, and allow to stand for 5 minutes. The colour produced is not more intense than the similarly prepared standard colour when viewed down the vertical axis of the tube in diffused light against a white background.

Standard colour

Measure 2 ml of iron standard FeTS and 40 ml of water into a comparison tube. Add 2 ml of citric acid (180 g/l) FeTS and 2 drops of mercaptoacetic acid R; mix, make alkaline with ammonia (~100 g/l) FeTS, dilute to 50 ml with water, and allow to stand for 5 minutes.

LIMIT TEST FOR ARSENIC

The limit test for arsenic is provided to demonstrate that the content of arsenic does not exceed the limit given in the individual monograph in terms of micrograms of arsenic per gram of the test substance.

To carry out the limit test for arsenic a solution is prepared from the test substance by a procedure specified in the monograph. This procedure assures that the solution in every case contains the whole of the arsenic (if any) present in the substance.

The standard stain against which the comparison is made contains 10 µg of As.

The procedure described may also be used to determine the amount of arsenic in the substance by matching the depth of colour of the stain with a series of standard stains. A stain equivalent to the 1 ml standard stain produced by operating on 10 g of a substance indicates that the amount of arsenic is 1 µg/g.

In the statements of arsenic limits, the permitted amount of arsenic is expressed as As.

Apparatus

A suitable type of apparatus is described below, though other acceptable constructions are available.

A wide-mouthed bottle of about 120 ml capacity, is fitted with a rubber bung through which passes a glass tube. The latter, made from ordinary glass tubing, has a total length of 200 mm and an internal diameter of exactly 6.5 mm (external diameter about 8 mm), is drawn out at one end to a diameter of about 1 mm, and has a hole not less than 2 mm in diameter blown in the side of the tube, near the constricted part. The tube is passed through the bung fitting the bottle so that, when inserted in the bottle containing 70 ml of liquid, the constricted end of the tube is above the surface of the liquid and the hole in the side is below the bottom of the bung. The upper end of the tube is cut off square, and is either slightly rounded off or ground smooth.

Two rubber bungs (about 25 mm × 25 mm), each with a hole bored centrally and true and exactly 6.5 mm in diameter, are fitted with a rubber band or spring clip for holding them tightly together. Alternatively, the two bungs may be replaced by any suitable construction satisfying the conditions of the test, as described below.

RECOMMENDED PROCEDURE

Pack the glass tube lightly with cotton-wool, previously moistened with lead acetate (80 g/l) TS and dried, so that the upper surface of the cotton-wool is not less than 25 mm below the top of the tube.

Insert the upper end of the tube into the narrow end of one of the pair of rubber bungs, either (1) to a depth of about 10 mm in the case of the tube with the rounded-off end or (2) so that the ground end of the tube is flush with the larger end of the bung. Place a piece of mercuric bromide paper AsR flat on the top of the bung, and place the other bung over it. Secure the assembly by means of a rubber band or spring clip, in such a manner that the borings of the two bungs (or the boring of the upper bung and the glass tube) meet to form a true tube 6.5 mm in diameter interrupted by a diaphragm of mercuric bromide paper AsR.

Instead of this method of attaching the mercuric bromide paper AsR, any other method may be used provided (1) that the whole of the evolved gas passes through the paper, (2) that the portion of the paper in contact with the gas is a circle 6.5 mm in diameter, and (3) that the paper is protected from sunlight during the test.

Place the solution, prepared as specified in the monograph, in the wide-mouthed bottle, add 1 g of potassium iodide AsR and 10 g of granulated zinc AsR, and place the prepared glass tube assembly quickly into position. Allow the reaction to proceed for 40 minutes. Compare any yellow stain that is produced on the mercuric bromide paper AsR, with a standard stain, produced in a similar manner with a known quantity of dilute arsenic AsTS. Make the comparison in daylight and immediately after simultaneous preparation of the test and standard stains; the stains fade on keeping.

The most suitable temperature for carrying out the test is generally about 40 °C but, as the rate of evolution of the gas varies somewhat with different batches of granulated zinc AsR, the temperature may be adjusted to obtain a regular, but not too violent, evolution of gas. The reaction may be accelerated by placing the apparatus on a warm surface, care being taken to ensure that the mercuric bromide paper AsR remains quite dry throughout the test.

Between successive tests, the tube must be washed with hydrochloric acid ($\sim$250 g/l) AsTS, rinsed with water, and dried.

Standard stain

Prepare a solution by adding 10 ml of stannated hydrochloric acid ($\sim$250 g/l) AsTS and 1 ml of dilute arsenic AsTS, to 50 ml of water. The resulting solution, when treated as described in the general test, yields a stain on the mercuric bromide paper AsR, referred to as the standard stain.

SULFATED ASH

RECOMMENDED PROCEDURE

Accurately weigh about 1 g of the substance, or the quantity specified in the monograph, into a suitable dish (usually platinum) and moisten with sulfuric acid ($\sim$1760 g/l) TS. Heat gently to remove the excess of acid and ignite at about 800 °C until all the black particles have disappeared; again moisten with sulfuric acid ($\sim$1760 g/l) TS and re-ignite. Add a small amount of ammonium carbonate R and ignite to constant weight.

OXYGEN FLASK METHOD

The oxygen flask method for the determination of halogens and sulfur in organic compounds consists of a combustion procedure followed by appropriate titrimetric determination. Combustion of the organic material in oxygen yields water-soluble inorganic products, which are determined as directed for the individual element.

Apparatus

The combustion is carried out in a suitable conical flask into the stopper of which is fused one end of a piece of platinum wire. A flask of 500 ml is used, unless otherwise specified in the monograph. Towards the other end of the wire, a piece of platinum gauze is attached to provide a means of holding the substance clear of the absorbing liquid during combustion.

RECOMMENDED PROCEDURES

CAUTION: The analyst should wear safety glasses and use a suitable safety shield between himself and the apparatus. The flask must be scrupulously clean and free from all traces of organic solvents.

Wrap the test substance in a piece of halide-free filter-paper about 5 cm long and 3 cm wide, secure the package in the platinum gauze, and insert one end of a narrow strip of filter-paper into it. Moisten the neck of the flask with water, place the specified absorbing liquid in the flask, fill the flask with oxygen, light the free end of the narrow strip of filter-paper and immediately insert the stopper. Hold the stopper firmly in place. When vigorous burning has begun, tilt the flask to prevent incompletely burned material falling into the liquid. Immediately after combustion is completed, shake the flask intermittently for 10 minutes, place a little water around the rim of the flask, carefully withdraw the stopper, and rinse the stopper, platinum wire, platinum gauze, and sides of the flask with water. Complete the analysis of this solution as specified in the monograph.

Pulverizable substances should be finely ground and thoroughly mixed before the specified quantity is weighed.

For liquids, use capsules of suitable material (e.g. methylcellulose). Place the specified quantity on about 15 mg of ashless filter-paper flock contained in one part of a capsule of suitable size, close the capsule, inserting one end of a narrow strip of filter-paper between the two parts, and secure the capsule in the platinum gauze.

Determination of bromine and chlorine

Using the oxygen flask method described above, burn the quantity of the substance specified in the monograph. The absorbing liquid consists of 17 ml of hydrogen peroxide ($\sim$60 g/l) TS and 3 ml of water. When the process is complete, rinse the stopper, platinum wire, platinum gauze, and sides of the flask with 40 ml of water.

Add 5 drops of bromophenol blue/ethanol TS and then, by drops, sodium hydroxide (0.1 mol/l) VS until the colour changes from yellow to blue. Then add 1 ml of nitric acid (3 g/l) TS and 5 drops of diphenylcarbazone/ethanol TS as indicator, and titrate with mercuric nitrate (0.01 mol/l) VS until the solution turns light violet.

Each ml of mercuric nitrate (0.01 mol/l) VS is equivalent to 1.598 mg of Br or 0.709 mg of Cl.

Determination of fluorine

Using the oxygen flask method described on p. 124, burn the quantity of the substance specified in the monograph. The absorbing liquid consists of 15 ml of water. When the process is complete, rinse the stopper, platinum wire, platinum gauze, and sides of the flask with 40 ml of water.

Add 0.6 ml of sodium alizarinsulfonate (1 g/l) TS and then, by drops, sodium hydroxide (0.1 mol/l) VS until the colour changes from pink to yellow. Add 5 ml of acetate buffer, pH 3.0, TS and titrate with thorium nitrate (0.005 mol/l) VS until the yellow colour changes to pinkish yellow.

Each ml of thorium nitrate (0.005 mol/l) VS is equivalent to 0.380 mg of F.

If a difficulty arises in observing the colour change of the indicator, a preliminary test with a solution containing known quantities of inorganic fluoride should be performed.

Determination of iodine

Using the oxygen flask method described on p. 124, burn the quantity of the substance specified in the monograph. The absorbing liquid consists of 10 ml of sodium hydroxide (0.2 mol/l) VS. When the process is complete, rinse the stopper, platinum wire, platinum gauze, and sides of the flask with 25 ml of potassium acetate TS to which 15 drops of bromine TS1 are added. Then rinse with 40 ml of water and add, by drops, formic acid (~1080 g/l) TS until discoloration, 20 ml of sulfuric acid (0.05 mol/l) VS, 0.5 g of potassium iodide R, and allow to stand for 5 minutes. Titrate the liberated iodine with sodium thiosulfate (0.05 mol/l) VS, adding starch TS as indicator towards the end of the titration.

Each ml of sodium thiosulfate (0.05 mol/l) VS is equivalent to 1.06 mg of I.

Determination of sulfur

Using the oxygen flask method described on p. 124, burn the quantity of the substance specified in the monograph. The absorbing liquid consists of 12.5 ml of hydrogen peroxide (~60 g/l) TS. When the process is complete, rinse the stopper, platinum wire, platinum gauze, and sides of the flask with 40 ml of water. Boil the solution for 10 minutes, cool, add 2 ml of acetic acid (~300 g/l) TS, and 20 ml of ethanol (~750 g/l) TS.

Titrate with barium nitrate (0.01 mol/l) VS using 2 drops of thorin (2 g/l) TS and 2 drops of methylthioninium chloride (0.2 g/l) TS as indicator until the yellow colour changes to pink.

Each ml of barium nitrate (0.01 mol/l) VS is equivalent to 0.321 mg of S.

COMPLEXOMETRIC TITRATIONS

Complexing agents of value as titrants are aminopolycarboxylic acids that possess the characteristic group

$$—N\begin{matrix} CH_2COOH \\ CH_2COOH \end{matrix}$$

Such compounds are capable of forming chelate complexes with many cations in which the cation is bound in a ring structure. The ring results from the formation of a salt-like bond between the cation and the carboxyl groups together with a coordinate bond through the lone pair of electrons of the nitrogen atom. If the ring is five-membered, the chelate thus formed is likely to have high stability, so the most useful chelating titrants are those that favour the formation of such rings. This is the case with edetic acid (ethylenediaminetetraacetic acid, EDTA); the commonly used disodium salt is known as disodium edetate. With most metals carrying more than unit positive charge, edetic acid forms highly water-soluble 1 : 1 complexes of such a structure that at least 3 five-membered chelate rings are formed, thus conferring high stability on the complex. In some cases, coordinate bonds other than those resulting from donation of the nitrogen lone pair of electrons may be formed with the carbonyl oxygens of the remaining carboxylic acid groups. Thus the complexes formed by calcium and by trivalent aluminium may be represented:

and

WHO 79051

The stability of such complexes is markedly dependent on pH. Most divalent metals form complexes that are stable in alkaline solution but alkaline earth chelates decompose below about pH 8, whereas many divalent metal complexes (zinc and lead, for example) are also stable in quite acid solution. Trivalent metal complexes, by virtue of the additional stability conferred by an increased number of chelate rings, are often stable even in strongly acid solutions. In alkaline solutions, however, some of these metals may be precipitated as hydroxides in the presence of edetic acid, not because of instability of the complex but because of the more powerful effect of the very low solubility product of the metal hydroxide.

Stability constants of the edetic acid chelates of some metals, as recorded by Schwarzenbach for 0.1 mol/l solutions at 20 °C are as follows:

Na	1.7
Li	2.8
Mg	8.7
Ca	10.6
Fe^{2+}	14.3
Al	15.5[a]
Zn	16.1
Pb	17.6
Hg^{2+}	20.4
Fe^{3+}	25.1

[a] The aluminium chelate is slow to form so that this metal is usually determined by back-titration.

In order to determine the equivalence point in titration of metal ions with edetic acid, it is necessary to use a suitable indicator that will react to the presence of free metal ions in solution. The indicator originally used by Schwarzenbach for titration of calcium ions was murexide (ammonium purpurate) but this is now rarely used. Perhaps the most widely used of indicators has been Mordant Black 11 (also known under several trade names). This has a blue colour in ammoniacal solution but yields red complexes with many metal ions in such solutions; the metal complexes so formed are generally weaker than the corresponding edetic acid complexes, so that titration with edetates will readily remove the metal from the indicator complex and a colour change to full blue signifies total titration of the metal present in solution. Mordant Black 11 is frequently used as a mixture with methyl orange, which serves to provide a screened (more readily detectable) endpoint.

Many other substances have been proposed and used as indicators for complexometric titrations, but the present discussion must be limited to a consideration of those that are of potential value in pharmaceutical applications. Calcon and calconcarboxylic acid give a very sharp colour change from wine-red to full blue when a calcium solution is titrated with sodium edetate in the pH range 12–14. If magnesium is present it is precipitated as hydroxide at this pH and, providing the alkali is added before the indicator, does not interfere. Neither of them, however, is very stable in alkaline solution and they should preferably be added at a late stage in the titration.

Another widely used indicator is xylenol orange; this is a conventional acid-base indicator into which iminodiacetic acid groups have been introduced, thus permitting the substance to act as a metal-complexing indicator. The indicator gives a clear colour change from pink-violet to yellow at the endpoint in titrations of aluminium, bismuth, lead, mercury, and zinc, and may be used from pH 2–6 according to the metal being titrated.

RECOMMENDED PROCEDURES

Aluminium

Dissolve the quantity of substance, accurately weighed, as specified in the monograph, in 2 ml of hydrochloric acid (1 mol/l) VS and 50 ml of water, unless other conditions of solution are given in the monograph. Add 50 ml of disodium edetate (0.05 mol/l) VS and neutralize to methyl red/ethanol TS with sodium hydroxide (1 mol/l) VS. Heat the solution to boiling and maintain in a boiling water-bath for at least 10 minutes, cool, add about 50 mg of xylenol orange indicator mixture R and 5 g of methenamine R and titrate the excess edetate with lead nitrate (0.05 mol/l) VS until the yellow solution turns pink-violet. Each ml of disodium edetate (0.05 mol/l) VS is equivalent to 1.349 mg of Al.

Bismuth

Dissolve the quantity of substance, accurately weighed, as specified in the monograph, in the minimum quantity of nitric acid (~130 g/l) TS, add 50 ml of water and adjust the pH to between 1 and 2 by dropwise addition of either nitric acid (~130 g/l) TS or ammonia (~100 g/l) TS. Add about 50 mg of xylenol orange indicator mixture R and slowly titrate with disodium ededate (0.05 mol/l) VS until the solution turns from pink-violet to a full yellow. Each ml of disodium edetate (0.05 mol/l) VS is equivalent to 10.45 mg of Bi.

Calcium

Dissolve the quantity of substance, accurately weighed, as specified in the monograph, in a few millilitres of water, acidified with a minimum quantity of hydrochloric acid (~70 g/l) TS if necessary, and then dilute to about 100 ml with water. Titrate with disodium edetate (0.05 mol/l) VS to within about 2 ml of the expected equivalence point, add 4 ml of sodium hydroxide (~300 g/l) TS and 0.1 g of calcon indicator mixture R or of calcon carboxylic acid indicator mixture R and continue the titration until the solution turns from pink to a full blue. Each ml of disodium edetate (0.05 mol/l) VS is equivalent to 2.004 mg of Ca.

Lead

Dissolve the quantity of substance, accurately weighed, as specified in the monograph, in 5–10 ml of water, acidified with a minimum quantity of acetic acid ($\sim$300 g/l) TS if necessary, and then dilute to about 50 ml with water. Add about 50 mg of xylenol orange indicator mixture R and sufficient methenamine R (about 5 g) to turn the solution red and titrate with disodium edetate (0.05 mol/l) VS until the solution turns from deep violet to full yellow. Each ml of disodium edetate (0.05 mol/l) VS is equivalent to 10.35 mg of Pb.

Magnesium

Dissolve the quantity of substance, accurately weighed, as specified in the monograph, in 5–10 ml of water, acidified with a minimum quantity of hydrochloric acid ($\sim$70 g/l) TS if necessary, and then dilute to about 50 ml with water. Add 10 ml of ammonium chloride buffer, pH 10.0, TS and 100 mg of Mordant Black 11 indicator mixture R and titrate with disodium edetate (0.05 mol/l) VS until the solution turns from violet to green. Each ml of disodium edetate (0.05 mol/l) VS is equivalent to 1.215 mg of Mg.

Zinc

Dissolve the quantity of substance, accurately weighed, as specified in the monograph, in 5–10 ml of water, acidified with a minimum quantity of acetic acid ($\sim$300 g/l) TS if necessary, and then dilute to about 50 ml with water. Add about 50 mg of xylenol orange indicator mixture R and sufficient methenamine R (about 5 g) to turn the solution red and titrate with disodium edetate (0.05 mol/l) VS until the solution turns from pink-violet to full yellow. Each ml of disodium edetate (0.05 mol/l) VS is equivalent to 3.268 mg of Zn.

NON-AQUEOUS TITRATION

Acids and bases have long been defined as substances that, when dissolved in water, furnish hydrogen and hydroxyl ions, respectively. This definition, introduced by Arrhenius, fails to recognize the fact that properties characteristic of acids or bases may be developed also in other solvents. A more generalized definition is that of Brönsted, who defined an acid as a proton donor, and a base as a proton acceptor.

Even broader is the definition of Lewis, who defined an acid as any material that will accept an electron pair, a base as any material that will donate an electron pair, and neutralization as the formation of a coordination bond between an acid and a base.

The apparent strength of an acid or base is determined by the extent of its reaction with a solvent. In aqueous solution all strong acids appear equally strong because they react with the solvent to undergo almost complete conversion to hydronium ion (H_3O^+) and the acid anion. In a weakly protophilic solvent such as acetic acid, the extent of formation of the acetonium ion ($CH_3COOH_2{}^+$) due to the addition of a proton provides a more sensitive differentiation of the strength of acids and shows that the order of decreasing strength for acids is perchloric, hydrobromic, sulfuric, hydrochloric, and nitric.

Acetic acid reacts incompletely with water to form hydronium ion and is, therefore, a weak acid. In contrast, it dissolves in a base such as ethylenediamine, and reacts so completely with the solvent that it behaves as a strong acid.

This so-called levelling effect is observed also for bases. In sulfuric acid almost all bases appear to be of the same strength. As the acid properties of the solvent decrease in the series sulfuric acid, acetic acid, phenol, water, pyridine and butylamine, bases dissolved in them become progressively weaker and the differences between bases are accentuated. In order of decreasing strength, strong bases of value for non-aqueous titrations are potassium methoxide, sodium methoxide, lithium methoxide, and tetrabutylammonium hydroxide.

Many water-insoluble compounds acquire enhanced acidic or basic properties when dissolved in organic solvents. Thus the choice of the appropriate solvent permits the determination of a variety of such materials by non-aqueous titration. Further, depending upon which part of a compound is physiologically active, it is often possible to titrate that part by proper selection of solvent and titrant. Pure compounds can be titrated directly, but it is often necessary to isolate the active ingredient in pharmaceutical preparations from interfering excipients and carriers.

The types of compounds that may be titrated as acids include acid halides, acid anhydrides, carboxylic acids, amino acids, enols such as barbiturates and xanthines, imides, phenols, pyrroles, and sulfonamides. The types of compounds that may be titrated as bases include amines, nitrogen-containing heterocyclic compounds, quarternary ammonium compounds, alkali salts of organic acids, alkali salts of inorganic acids, and some salts of amines. Many salts of halogen acids may be titrated in acetic acid or acetic anhydride after the addition of mercuric acetate, which removes halide ion as the unionized mercuric halide complex. In the case of hydrochlorides of weak bases not containing acetylatable groupings it is also possible to titrate in acetic anhydride without the addition of mercuric acetate and using an indicator such as malachite green or crystal violet. Titrations carried out in the presence of an excess of acetic anhydride must be applied cautiously, however, since any reaction of the anhydride with the substance being titrated may give rise to low results.

In the titration of a basic compound, a volumetric solution of perchloric acid in glacial acetic acid is usually used, although perchloric acid in dioxan may be useful in special cases. In the titration of an acidic compound, a volumetric solution of lithium methoxide in a methanol-toluene solvent is often used. For many applications it is convenient to use a solution of tetrabutylammonium hydroxide in toluene; sodium methoxide, formerly in wide use, may often give rise to troublesome gelatinous precipitates.

Because of interference by carbon dioxide, solvents for acidic compounds must be protected from excessive exposure to the atmosphere by a suitable cover or by an inert atmosphere during the titration. A blank determination should be carried out and the volume generally should not exceed 0.01 ml of a 0.1 mol/l titrant for each ml of solvent.

The endpoint may be determined visually by colour change, or potentiometrically. If the calomel reference electrode is used, it is advantageous to replace the aqueous potassium chloride solution in the salt bridge with lithium perchlorate/acetic acid TS for titrations in acidic solvents, or potassium chloride in methanol for titrations in basic solvents. It should be recognized that certain indicators in common use (crystal violet, for example) undergo a series of colour changes and, in establishing a non-aqueous titration method for a particular use, care should be taken to ensure that the colour change specified as the endpoint of the titration corresponds to the maximum value of dE/dV (where E is the electromotive force and V the volume of titrant) in a potentiometric titration of the substance under consideration.

When using titrants prepared with solvents that may have a relatively high coefficient of expansion, for example glacial acetic acid, toluene etc., care should be taken to compensate for differences in temperature that may exist between the time the titrant is used and that at which it was standardized.

RECOMMENDED PROCEDURES

Method A (for bases and their salts)

Prepare a solution as specified in the monograph or dissolve the substance being examined in a suitable volume of glacial acetic acid Rl, previously neutralized to crystal violet/acetic acid TS, warming and cooling if necessary. Alternatively the titration blank for the solvent and indicator may be established in a separate determination. When the substance is a salt of a hydrohalic acid, add 10 ml of mercuric acetate/acetic acid TS. When the endpoint is determined visually by colour change, add 2–3 drops of crystal violet/acetic acid TS, and titrate with perchloric acid of the specified concentration (mol/l) to the appropriate colour change of the indicator. When a different indicator is specified in the monograph, this indicator should also be used for the neutralization of the glacial acetic acid Rl, and mercuric acetate/acetic acid TS, and the standardization of the titrant.

When the equivalence point is determined potentiometrically, the indicator is omitted and neutralization of the solution and standardization of the titrant are also carried out potentiometrically. A glass electrode and a saturated calomel cell (containing potassium chloride (350 g/l) TS) as reference electrode, are used. The junction between the calomel electrode and the titration liquid should have a reasonably low electrical resistance and there should be a minimum of transfer of liquid from one side to the other. Serious instability may result unless the connexions between the potentiometer and the electrode system are in accordance with the manufacturer's instructions.

When the temperature (t_2) at which the titration is carried out differs from the temperature (t_1) at which the titrant was standardized, multiply the volume of the titrant required by $[1 + 0.001(t_1 - t_2)]$ and calculate the result of the assay from the corrected volume.

Method B (for acids)

The titrant, solvent and (in the case where the endpoint is determined visually) the indicator to be used for each substance, are specified in the monograph.

Protect the solution and titrant from carbon dioxide of the atmosphere throughout the determination. This may conveniently be done by replacing the air above the titration liquid with nitrogen.

Dissolve the substance being examined in a suitable volume of the solvent previously neutralized to the indicator, warming and cooling if necessary, or prepare a solution as specified in the monograph. Titrate to the appropriate colour change of the indicator. Carry out a blank determination and make any necessary corrections. The titrant is standardized using the same solvent and indicator as specified for the substance.

When the equivalence point is established potentiometrically, the indicator is omitted and neutralization of the solution and standardization of the titrant are also carried out potentiometrically.

A glass electrode and a saturated calomel reference electrode in which the aqueous potassium chloride (350 g/l) TS has been replaced by a saturated solution of potassium chloride R in methanol R, are used. The junction between the calomel electrode and the titration liquid should have a reasonably low electrical resistance and there should be a minimum of transfer of the liquid from one side to the other. Serious instability may result unless the connexions between the potentiometer and the electrode system are made in accordance with the manufacturer's instruction.

NITRITE TITRATION

Nitrite titration is a titration method used particularly for the assay of primary aromatic amines.

The apparatus usually used in an electrometric procedure for nitrite titration is composed of an open titration vessel containing two platinum electrodes connected to a suitable circuit. The electrodes should have a potential difference of 50–100 mV. The circuit should include a device for measuring current with a sensitivity of 0.1 to 1 nA, usually with an indicating needle. The titration vessel should be provided with a suitable mechanical or magnetic stirring device, or a stream of nitrogen passing through the solution may be used to mix this solution. Electrodes made of platinum wire 0.5 mm in diameter and about 20 mm long are suitable. Before each use, the electrodes should be cleaned by immersing them for a few seconds in boiling nitric acid ($\sim$1000 g/l) TS, to which about 1 mg/ml of ferric chloride R has previously been added, and then thoroughly rinsing them with water.

RECOMMENDED PROCEDURE

Place 20 ml of hydrochloric acid ($\sim$250 g/l) TS and 50 ml of water in the titration vessel, add the quantity of the test substance and, if indicated, a catalyst, as specified in the monograph and stir to dissolve; cool to about 15 °C and titrate slowly with sodium nitrite (0.1 mol/l) VS, placing the burette tip below the surface of the solution. During the addition of the titrant, stir the solution continuously and gently, without pulling a vortex of air under the surface, and maintain the temperature of the solution at about 15 °C.

When the titration is within 1 ml of the estimated endpoint, add the titrant in 0.1 ml portions, allowing not less than 1 minute to elapse before adding subsequent portions. Initially, the needle of the measuring device deflects at every addition of reagent and then returns to its original position. No deflexion is observed when the endpoint of the determination is reached.

DETERMINATION OF WATER
BY THE KARL FISCHER METHOD

The titrimetric determination of water by the Karl Fischer method depends on the reaction that takes place quantitatively between water and a reagent consisting of sulfur dioxide and iodine in anhydrous pyridine and usually methanol. The reaction is carried out in a suitable solvent such as methanol or acetic acid.

The reagents and solutions used in the determination of water by this method are sensitive to water and precautions must be taken throughout to prevent exposure to atmospheric moisture.

The titration vessel is fitted with two platinum electrodes, a gas inlet tube if needed, a stopper, which accommodates the burette tip, and a vent tube protected by a desiccant. The substance to be titrated is introduced through an inlet tube or side-arm, which can be closed by an airtight stopper. The Karl Fischer reagent TS is protected from light and stored in a bottle into which is fitted an automatic burette. The reagent is pumped into the burette by means of a hand bellows, the access of moisture being prevented by a suitable arrangement of desiccant tubes. Stirring is accomplished magnetically or by means of a stream of suitably dried nitrogen passed through the solution during the titration.

The endpoint is obtained by using an electrical circuit composed of a microammeter, platinum electrodes, and a 1.5-V or 2-V battery connected across a variable resistance of about 2000 Ω. The resistance is adjusted so that an initial current passes through the platinum electrodes in series with a microammeter. After each addition of reagent, the pointer of the microammeter is deflected but quickly returns to its original position. At the end of the reaction a deflexion is obtained that persists for 10–15 seconds. Alternatively, the endpoint can also be determined by a voltametric method. A potential difference of 30–50 mV is applied to the platinum electrodes to serve as a constant polarizing current and the solution is titrated with the reagent. The potential difference is monitored by means of a microvoltmeter. The endpoint is reached when the voltmeter indicates a stable decrease of voltage. In the voltametric method the endpoint may also be obtained graphically by plotting the voltage versus the volume of the reagent, and establishing the beginning of the drop in potential.

Direct titration (Method A)

Add about 20 ml of dehydrated methanol R, unless otherwise specified in the monograph, to the titration vessel and titrate to the endpoint with Karl Fischer reagent TS. Quickly transfer the specified quantity of substance, accurately weighed, to the titration vessel. Stir for 1 minute and titrate again to the endpoint with Karl Fischer reagent TS.

Backtitration (Method B)

Add about 10 ml of dehydrated methanol R, unless otherwise specified in the monograph, to the titration vessel and titrate to the endpoint with Karl Fischer reagent TS. Quickly transfer the specified quantity of substance, accurately weighed, to the titration vessel, followed by an accurately measured amount of Karl Fischer reagent TS, sufficient to give an excess of about 1 ml. Allow to stand protected from light for 1 minute or the time specified in the monograph, stirring from time to time.

Titrate the excess of Karl Fischer reagent TS to the endpoint with dehydrated methanol R, to which has been added an accurately known amount of water, usually equivalent to about 2.5 mg/ml.

DETERMINATION OF METHOXYL

The contents of methoxy-groups in an organic substance are assayed by reacting the substance with concentrated hydriodic acid; methyl iodide produced in the reaction is distilled off, absorbed into a suitable absorbing liquid, and its amount determined titrimetrically.

Apparatus

The apparatus consists of a 25-ml round-bottomed boiling flask into which is sealed a capillary side-arm, 1 mm in diameter, to provide an inlet for a stream of carbon dioxide. The flask is also fitted with an air condenser, approximately 25 cm in height and about 9 mm in internal diameter. A suitable scrubber device containing about 2 ml of water is placed over the condenser. Add 5 ml of antimony sodium tartrate (50 g/l) TS to the scrubber. The outlet from the scrubber terminates in a tube that dips below the surface of the absorbing liquid in the first of two receivers connected in series. For greater convenience in use and cleaning, separate parts of the apparatus are connected by means of ground glass conical or ball joints.

RECOMMENDED PROCEDURE

Place a quantity of the substance being tested, accurately weighed, as specified in the monograph, in the boiling flask with a boiling rod. Add 2.5 ml of melted phenol R and 5 ml of hydriodic acid ($\sim$970 g/l) TS, and connect the flask to the condenser. Add potassium acetate TS to each of the two receivers, about 6 ml to the first one and about 4 ml to the second, and to each receiver 6 drops of bromine R. Pass a slow uniform stream of carbon dioxide R through the capillary side-arm of the boiling flask, and heat the liquid gently by means of a mantled microburner or another suitable device, at such a rate that the vapours of the boiling liquid rise halfway up the condenser. For most substances 30 minutes are sufficient to complete the reaction and sweep out the apparatus. Wash the contents of both receivers into a 250-ml conical flask containing 5 ml of sodium acetate (150 g/l) TS.

Adjust the volume of the liquid to approximately 125 ml, and add 6 drops of formic acid ($\sim$1080 g/l) TS. Rotate the flask until the colour due to the bromine is discharged, then add 12 drops of formic acid ($\sim$1080 g/l) TS, stopper the flask and mix the contents thoroughly so as to remove any free bromine including the vapour above the liquid, and allow the solution to stand for 1–2 minutes; add 1 g of potassium iodide R and 5 ml of sulfuric acid ($\sim$100 g/l) TS, and titrate the liberated iodine with sodium thiosulfate (0.1 mol/l) VS using starch TS as indicator. Repeat the operation without the substance being tested, and deduct the volume of sodium thiosulfate (0.1 mol/l) VS used from the volume required in the determination of methoxyl.

Each ml of sodium thiosulfate (0.1 mol/l) VS is equivalent to 0.5172 mg of methoxyl (CH_3O).

DETERMINATION OF NITROGEN

RECOMMENDED PROCEDURES

Procedure for macrodetermination (Method A)

Place the amount of test substance specified in the monograph in a 200-ml long-necked flask, add 1 g of a mixture composed of 10 parts of potassium sulfate R or anhydrous sodium sulfate R and 1 part of copper(II) sulfate R, followed by nitrogen-free sulfuric acid ($\sim$1760 g/l) TS, using the quantities of the substance and of sulfuric acid specified in the monograph. Heat the mixture over a small flame until a clear green solution is obtained and boil gently for a further 30 minutes unless otherwise specified in the monograph; precautions should be taken to prevent the upper part of the flask from becoming overheated. Cool, dilute to 75–85 ml with water, using suitable precautions, and add a piece of granulated zinc R and a solution of 15 g of sodium hydroxide R and 2 g of sodium thiosulfate R in 25 ml of water. The quantity of sodium hydroxide should be increased, if necessary, to ensure that, before distillation, the mixture is strongly alkaline. Immediately connect the flask to a distillation apparatus, mix the contents, distil the liberated ammonia into 16 ml of boric acid (50 g/l) TS, and titrate with sulfuric acid (0.05 mol/l) VS using methyl red/ethanol TS as indicator. Repeat the operation without the substance being tested; the difference between the titrations represents the ammonia liberated by the substance being tested. Each ml of sulfuric acid (0.05 mol/l) VS is equivalent to 1.401 mg of N.

Procedure for microdetermination (Method B)

Place the amount of test substance specified in the monograph in a suitable digestion tube, add 3 drops of copper(II) sulfate (190 g/l) TS and 1 ml of nitrogen-free sulfuric acid ($\sim$1760 g/l) TS and boil gently for 10 minutes; cool; add 1 g of anhydrous sodium sulfate R and 10 mg of selenium R, boil gently for 1 hour and cool. Transfer the contents of the digestion tube to (or attach it to) an ammonia microdistillation apparatus, add 6 ml of sodium hydroxide ($\sim$400 g/l) TS and pass steam through the flask; distil for 7 minutes, collecting the distillate in a mixture of 5 ml of boric acid (50 g/l) TS, 5 ml of water, and 1 drop of methyl red/methylthioninium chloride TS and titrate with hydrochloric acid (0.015 mol/l) VS. Repeat the operation without the substance being tested; the difference between the titrations represents the ammonia liberated by the substance being tested. Each ml of hydrochloric acid (0.015 mol/l) VS is equivalent to 0.210 mg of N.

DETERMINATION OF IODINE VALUE

The iodine value of a substance is the weight of halogens expressed as iodine absorbed by 100 parts by weight of the substance. The quantity of substance used in the determination should be such that at least 70 % of the iodine added, as provided in the recommended procedure, is not absorbed. Unless otherwise specified in the monograph, the quantity of the substance indicated in the following table should be used for the determination, depending on the expected iodine value:

Iodine value	Quantity of substance in g
less than 20	1.0
20 — 60	0.5 — 0.25
60 — 100	0.25 — 0.15
more than 100	0.15 — 0.10

RECOMMENDED PROCEDURE

Place a quantity of the test substance, accurately weighed, as specified in the monograph, in a dry 300-ml to 500-ml stoppered flask, add 15 ml of carbon tetrachloride R and dissolve. Add 25 ml of iodine bromide TS, insert the stopper, previously moistened with potassium iodide (80 g/l) TS, shake the flask gently, and keep in the dark for 30 minutes, unless otherwise specified in the monograph. Add 20 ml of potassium iodide (80 g/l) TS and 150 ml of water, and, whilst shaking the contents of the flask, titrate with sodium thiosulfate (0.1 mol/l) VS, adding starch TS as indicator towards the end of the titration. Note the number of ml required (a). At the same time carry out the operation in exactly the same manner, but without the substance being tested, and note the number of ml of sodium thiosulfate (0.1 mol/l) VS required (b). Calculate the iodine value from the following formula:

$$\text{Iodine value} = \frac{(b - a) \times 0.01269 \times 100}{\text{weight (in g) of substance}}$$

DETERMINATION OF PEROXIDES IN FIXED OILS

RECOMMENDED PROCEDURE

Dissolve the quantity of test substance as specified in the monograph, usually about 3 g, accurately weighed, in 15 ml of chloroform R and 30 ml of glacial acetic acid R in a 250-ml glass-stoppered flask. Add 1 ml of a freshly prepared solution of 1.3 g of potassium iodide R in 1 ml of water, stopper the flask, mix by gentle swirling and set aside in the dark for 3 minutes. Add 100 ml of water, shake, and titrate with sodium thiosulfate (0.01 mol/l) VS, using starch TS as indicator. Repeat the operation without the substance being tested and calculate the difference between the titrations, the limit value being specified in the monograph.

DETERMINATION OF SAPONIFICATION VALUE

The saponification value is the number of mg of potassium hydroxide required to neutralize the fatty acids resulting from the complete hydrolysis of 1 g of the substance.

In the procedure described, a 50-ml burette should preferably be used for titration, as in the blank titration the volume of hydrochloric acid (0.5 mol/l) VS used is exactly 35.5 ml when the concentration of ethanolic potassium hydroxide is exactly 40 g/l.

RECOMMENDED PROCEDURE

Place about 2 g of the test substance, accurately weighed, or the quantity specified in the monograph, in a flask with a capacity of about 200 ml, add 25 ml of potassium hydroxide/ethanol, TS1 attach a reflux condenser, and heat in a boiling water-bath for 30 minutes, or the time specified in the monograph, frequently rotating the contents of the flask; immediately add 1 ml of phenolphthalein/ethanol TS and titrate the excess of alkali with hydrochloric acid (0.5 mol/l) VS. Note the number of ml of hydrochloric acid (0.5 mol/l) VS required to titrate the sample (a). Repeat the operation without the substance being tested and note the number of ml of hydrochloric acid (0.5 mol/l) VS required for neutralization (b). Calculate the saponification value from the following formula:

$$\text{Saponification value} = \frac{(b - a) \times 0.02805 \times 1000}{\text{weight (in g) of substance}}$$

DETERMINATION OF UNSAPONIFIABLE MATTER

The term "unsaponifiable matter" refers to those substances present in oils or fats that are not saponified by alkali hydroxides and are extractable into ether.

RECOMMENDED PROCEDURE

Place a quantity of the test substance, accurately weighed, as specified in the monograph, in a flask provided with a reflux condenser and boil in a water-bath for 1 hour with 25 ml of potassium hydroxide/ethanol (0.5 mol/l) VS, with frequent swirling of contents. Wash the contents of the flask into a separator by means of 50 ml of water and, while the liquid is still slightly warm, extract by shaking vigorously with 3 successive quantities, each of 50 ml, of ether R, washing out the flask with the first quantity of ether R. (CAUTION: Ether should be free of peroxides.) Take care to release frequently and carefully the pressure that may build up inside the separator. Combine the ethereal solutions in another separator containing 20 ml of water. (If the ethereal solutions contain solid suspended matter, filter them into the separator through a fat-free filter-paper and wash the filter-paper with ether R). Gently rotate the separator for a few minutes without violent shaking, allow the liquids to separate, and run off the aqueous layer. Wash the ethereal solution by shaking vigorously with 2 successive quantities, each of 20 ml, of water; then treat 3 times with 20 ml of potassium hydroxide (0.5 mol/l) VS (NOTE: aqueous reagent), shaking vigorously on each occasion and washing with 20 ml of water after each treatment. Finally wash with successive quantities, each of 20 ml, of water until the aqueous layer is no longer alkaline to phenolphthalein/ethanol TS. Transfer the ethereal extract to a weighed flask, washing out the separator with ether R; distil off the ether with the necessary precautions and add 3 ml of acetone R.

By the aid of a gentle current of air remove the solvent completely from the flask, which is preferably held obliquely and rotated, almost entirely immersed, in a water-bath at about 60 °C. Dry to constant weight at a temperature not above 80 °C and dissolve the contents of the flask in 10 ml of ethanol (~750 g/l) TS, previously neutralized to phenolphthalein/ethanol TS. Titrate with carbonate-free sodium hydroxide (0.1 mol/l) VS, using phenolphthalein/ethanol TS as indicator. If the amount of carbonate-free sodium hydroxide (0.1 mol/l) required does not exceed 0.2 ml, the amount weighed is to be taken as the unsaponifiable matter. Calculate the unsaponifiable matter as a percentage of the oil or fat. If the amount of carbonate-free sodium hydroxide (0.1 mol/l) VS required exceeds 0.2 ml, the amount weighed cannot be taken as the unsaponifiable matter and the test must be repeated.

DETERMINATION OF ACID VALUE

The acid value is the number of mg of potassium hydroxide required to neutralize the free acid in 1 g of the substance.

RECOMMENDED PROCEDURE

Accurately weigh about 10 g of the substance, or the quantity specified in the monograph, into a 250-ml flask, and add 50 ml of a mixture of equal volumes of ethanol (~750 g/l) TS and ether R, which has been neutralized with potassium hydroxide (0.1 mol/l) VS after the addition of 1 ml of phenolphthalein/ethanol TS. Heat, if necessary, until the substance has completely dissolved, cool; titrate with potassium hydroxide (0.1 mol/l) VS, constantly shaking the contents of the flask until a pink colour, which persists for 15 seconds, is obtained. Note the number of ml required (a). Calculate the acid value from the following formula:

$$\text{Acid value} = \frac{a \times 0.00561 \times 1000}{\text{weight (in g) of substance}}$$

BIOLOGICAL METHODS

MICROBIOLOGICAL ASSAY OF ANTIBIOTICS

The potency (activity) of an antibiotic product is expressed as the ratio of the dose that inhibits the growth of a suitable susceptible microorganism to the dose of an International Biological Standard, an International Biological Reference Preparation, or an International Chemical Reference Substance of that antibiotic that produces similar inhibition. Properly validated secondary reference materials may also be utilized in the assay. To carry out the assay a comparison is made between the inhibition of the growth of microorganisms produced by known concentrations of the reference material and that produced by measured dilutions of the test substance. This response can be measured by the diffusion method, as described below, or in a liquid medium by the turbidimetric method.

An International Unit is the specific activity contained in such an amount (weight) of the relevant International Biological Standard or International Biological Reference Preparation as the WHO Expert Committee on Biological Standardization may from time to indicate as the quantity exactly equivalent to the unit accepted for international use. In some cases, when owing to the properties of the material, difficulties are experienced in weighing with adequate accuracy small amounts of the relevant International Biological Standard or International Biological Reference Preparation, international units are defined on the basis of the total contents of the material in an ampoule or a vial. A defined number of international units is then assigned to the total contents of an ampoule or a vial; this material has to be carefully removed with an appropriate solvent and the final volume of the solution has to be accurately adjusted.

International Chemical Reference Substances do not have defined units of biological activity. The potency of those products for which biological assays are required are in such cases expressed in terms of an equivalent weight of the pure substance.

RECOMMENDED PROCEDURE

Use Petri dishes or rectangular trays filled to a depth of 3–4 mm, unless otherwise indicated in the monograph, with a culture medium that has previously been inoculated with a suitable inoculum of a susceptible test organism prepared as described below. The nutrient agar may be composed of two separate layers of which only the upper one may be inoculated. The concentration of the inoculum should be so selected that the sharpest zones of inhibition and suitable dose response at different concentrations of the standard are obtained. When using the inoculum prepared as described below, an inoculated medium containing 1 ml of inoculum per 100 ml of the culture medium is usually suitable.   When the inoculum consists of a suspension of vegetative organisms, the temperature of the molten agar medium must not exceed 48–50 °C at the time of inoculation.   The dishes or trays should be specially selected with flat bottoms.   During the filling they should be placed on a flat, horizontal surface so as to ensure that the layer of the medium will be of a uniform thickness.   With some test organisms, the procedure may be improved if the inoculated plates are allowed to dry for 30 minutes at room temperature before use, or refrigerated at 4 °C for several hours.

For the application of the test solution, small sterile cylinders of uniform size, approximately 10 mm high and having an internal diameter of approximately 5 mm, made of suitable material such as glass, porcelain, or stainless steel, are placed on the surface of the inoculated medium. Instead of cylinders, holes 8–10 mm in diameter may be bored in the medium with a previously sterilized borer.   Other methods of application of the test solution may also be used.   The arrangement on the plate should be such that overlapping of zones is avoided.

Solutions of the reference material of known concentration and corresponding dilutions of the test substance, presumed to be of approximately the same concentration, are prepared in a sterile buffer of a suitable pH value.   To assess the validity of the assay at least 3 different doses of the reference material should be used together with an equal number of doses of the test substance having the same presumed activity as the solutions of the reference material.   The dose levels used should be in geometric progression, for example, by preparing a series of dilutions in the ratio 2 : 1.   Once the relationship between the logarithm of concentration of the antibiotic and the diameter of the zone of inhibition has been shown to be approximately rectilinear for the system used, routine assays may be carried out using only 2 concentrations of the reference material and 2 dilutions of the test substance.   Where a monograph gives directions for the initial preparation of a solution of the substance, this solution is then diluted as necessary with the appropriate sterile buffer.

The solutions of the reference material and the test substance are preferably arranged in the form of a Latin square when rectangular trays are employed.   When Petri dishes are used, the solutions are arranged on each dish so that the solutions of the reference material and those of the test substance alternate around the dish and are placed in such a manner that the highest concentrations of the reference material and of the test substance are not adjacent.   The solutions are placed in the cylinders or holes by means of a pipette that delivers a uniform volume of liquid. When the holes are used the delivered volume should be sufficient to fill them almost completely.

The plates are incubated at a suitable temperature, the selected temperature being controlled at ± 0.5 °C, for approximately 16 hours, and the diameters or areas of the zones of inhibition produced by the varied concentrations of the standard and of the test substance are measured accurately, preferably to the nearest 0.1 mm of the actual zone size, by using a suitable measuring device. From the results, the potency of the tested substance is calculated. Suitable publications on the statistics of bioassays are listed below.

Conditions for the assay of individual antibiotics and suitable test organisms are given in the monographs. The choice of an appropriate strain of test organism may be critical for the assay. For easy reference, examples of suitable test organisms for a number of antibiotics are shown in Table 4. The designations of the test strains are as follows:

NCTC — National Collection of Type Cultures, Central Public Health Laboratory, Colindale, London, England

NCYC — National Collection of Yeast Cultures, Brewing Industry Research Foundation, Nutfield, Redhill, Surrey, England

ATCC — American Type Culture Collection, Rockville, Maryland 20852, USA

Other suitable strains of test organisms can be used. Additional information regarding sources of suitable strains may be obtained from Biologicals, World Health Organization, Geneva, Switzerland.

Precision of the assay

In order to determine whether or not a substance satisfies the requirements for potency specified in the monograph, the assay should, if necessary, be repeated until the required precision has been attained. This precision is such that the fiducial limits (P = 0.95) of the mean estimated potency, expressed as a percentage of the mean estimated potency, should be within the required range given in the individual monographs.

Calculation of results

The following publications contain suitable methods that may be used to carry out the statistical evaluation of the microbiological assay of antibiotics:

1. *Specifications for the quality control of pharmaceutical publications (Second edition of the International Pharmacopoeia)*, Geneva, World Health Organization, 1967, Appendix 45: *Biological assays and tests.*
2. C.I. BLISS: *Statistics of bioassay*, New York, Academic Press, 1952.
3. C.I. BLISS: *Statistics in biology*, vol. I, New York, McGraw Hill, 1967.
4. C.I. BLISS: *Statistics in biology*, vol. II, New York, McGraw Hill, 1970.

5. D.J. FINNEY: *Statistical methods in biological assays*, London, Griffin, 1964.

6. W. HEWITT: *Microbiological assay*, New York, Academic Press, 1977.

7. J. PHILIPPE: *Les methodes statistiques en pharmacie et en chimie*, Paris, Masson, 1967.

The methods of carrying out the statistical evaluation of the micro-biological assay of antibiotics are also described in many national and regional pharmacopoeias.

TABLE 4. TEST ORGANISMS AND CONDITIONS OF ASSAY OF INDIVIDUAL ANTIBIOTICS

Antibiotic	Test organism	Culture medium; final pH	Phosphate buffer, sterile, pH[a], TS	Concentration (weight or International Units per ml)[b]	Incubation temperature (in °C)
Bacitracin	*Micrococcus luteus* NCTC 7743; ATCC 10240	Cm1; 7.0–7.1	7.0	1–4 IU	35–37
	Micrococcus luteus NCTC 7743; ATCC 10240	Cm1; 6.5–6.6	6.0	1–4 IU	30–31
Cefalexin	*Staphylococcus aureus* NCTC 6571; ATCC 9144	Cm1; 6.5–6.6	6.0	10–40 µg	32–35
	Staphylococcus aureus ATCC 6538-P	Cm1; 6.5–6.6	6.0	10–40 µg	32–35
Cefalotin	*Staphylococcus aureus* NCTC 6571; ATCC 9144	Cm1; 6.5–6.6	6.0	0.5–2 IU	32–35
	Staphylococcus aureus ATCC 6538-P	Cm1; 6.5–6.6	6.0	0.5–2 IU	32–35
Chlortetracycline	*Bacillus pumilus* NCTC 8241; ATCC 14884	Cm1; 6.5–6.6	4.5	2–20 IU	37–39
	Bacillus cereus ATCC 11778	Cm1; 5.9–6.0	4.5	0.05–0.2 IU	30-33
Cloxacillin	*Bacillus subtilis* NCTC 8236; ATCC 11774	Cm1; 6.5–6.6	7.0	5–20 µg	37–39
	Staphylococcus aureus ATCC 6538-P	Cm1; 6.5–6.6	6.0	2–8 µg	32–35
Dicloxacillin	*Staphylococcus aureus* NCTC 6571; ATCC 9144	Cm1; 6.6	6.0	2.5–10 µg	37–39
	Staphylococcus aureus ATCC 6538-P	Cm1; 6.5–6.6	6.0	2–8 µg	32–35
Erythromycin	*Bacillus pumilus* NCTC 8241; ATCC 14884	Cm1; 8.0–8.1	8.0	5–25 IU	37–39
	Micrococcus luteus ATCC 9341	Cm1; 8.0–8.1	8.0	0.5–1.5 IU	35–37

Antibiotic	Test organism	Culture medium; final pH	Phosphate buffer, sterile, pH^a, TS	Concentration (weight or International Units per ml)^b	Incubation temperature (in °C)
Neomycin	Bacillus pumilus NCTC 8241; ATCC 14884	Cm1; 8.0–8.1	8.0	2–14 IU	37–39
	Staphylococcus aureus ATCC 6538-P	Cm1; 7.8-8.0	8.0	2–20 IU	35–37
	Staphylococcus epidermidis ATCC 12228	Cm1; 8.0–8.1	8.0	0.5–2 IU	35–37
Novobiocin	Bacillus subtilis NCTC 10315;	Cm1; 6.5–6.6	6.0	1–5 IU	30–33
	Micrococcus luteus ATCC 9341	Cm1; 6.5–6.6	6.0	10–50 IU	30–35
Nystatin	Saccharomyces cerevisiae NCYC 87; ATCC 9763	Cm3; 6.0–6.2	—^{c}	25–300 IU	35–37
Oxacillin	Bacillus subtilis NCTC 8236; ATCC 11774	Cm1; 6.5–6.6	7.0	2.5–10 µg	37–39
	Staphylococcus aureus ATCC 6538-P	Cm1; 6.5–6.6	6.0	2–8 µg	32–35
Oxytetracycline	Bacillus pumilus NCTC 8241; ATCC 14884	Cm1; 6.5–6.6	4.5	2–20 IU	37–39
	Bacillus cereus ATCC 11778	Cm1; 5.9–6.0	4.5	0.5–2 IU	30–33
Polymyxin B	Bordetella bronchiseptica NCTC 8344; ATCC 4617	Cm2; 7.2–7.3	6.0, TS3	20–100 IU	35–37
	Bordetella bronchiseptica NCTC 8344; ATCC 4617	Cm2; 7.2–7.3	7.2	50–200 IU	35–37
	Escherichia coli ATCC 10536	Cm1; 6.5–6.6	7.2	5–100 IU	35–37
Streptomycin	Bacillus subtilis NCTC 8236; ATCC 11774	Cm1; 7.9–8.0	8.0	5–20 IU	37–39
	Bacillus subtilis ATCC 6633	Cm1; 8.0–8.1	8.0	3–15 IU	35–37
Tetracycline	Bacillus pumilus NCTC 8241; ATCC 14884	Cm1; 6.5–6.6	4.5	2–20 IU	37–39
	Bacillus cereus ATCC 11778	Cm1; 5.9–6.0	4.5	0.5–2 IU	30–33

^{a} Phosphate buffers, sterile, of suitable pH. Buffers designated as TS, TS1, or TS2 may be used.
^{b} Range within which suitable concentrations may be found.
^{c} The preparation of the solution of the reference material and of the corresponding dilution of the test substance is done as described in the monograph with the aid of dimethylformamide R and phosphate buffer, sterile, pH 6.0 TS3.

Culture media

The formulae for the culture media (Cm) referred to in Table 4 are described in "List of reagents, test solutions and volumetric solutions" (see page 175). In each instance the final pH is adjusted to that stated in the table.

Preparation of inoculum

Bacillus cereus; Bacillus pumilus; Bacillus subtilis. The test organism is grown for 7 days at a temperature of 37–39 °C on the surface of culture medium Cm1 (pH 6.5–6.6 after sterilization) to which has been added 1 μg of manganese sulfate R per ml. Using sterile water, the growth, which consists mainly of spores, is washed off, heated for 30 minutes at 70 °C, and suitably diluted — for example, to give between 10^7 and 10^8 spores per ml. The spore suspension may be stored for long periods at a temperature not exceeding 4 °C.

Bordetella bronchiseptica. The test organism is grown overnight on culture medium Cm2 (pH 6.5–6.6 after sterilization) at a temperature of 35–37 °C. A suspension is prepared by washing off the growth and diluting with sterile water or saline TS to a suitable opacity, for example, such that a 1-cm layer transmits 50 % of the incident light when examined at 650 nm. The suspension may be stored for up to 2 weeks at a temperature not exceeding 4 °C.

A freshly prepared inoculum may be replaced by a suitable suspension of the inoculum in a suitable vehicle, such as sterile peptone (1 g/l) TS2 that has been stored frozen at −70 °C and subsequently thawed.

Micrococcus luteus. The test organism is grown overnight on culture medium Cm1 (pH 6.5–6.6 after sterilization) at a temperature of 35–37 °C. A suspension is prepared by washing off the growth and diluting with saline TS to a suitable opacity, for example, such that a 1-cm layer of a 1 in 50 dilution transmits 80 % of the incident light when examined at 650 nm. The suspension may be stored for up to 2 weeks at a temperature not exceeding 4 °C.

A freshly prepared inoculum may be replaced by a suitable suspension of the inoculum in a suitable vehicle, such as sterile peptone (1 g/l) TS2 that has been stored frozen at −70 °C and subsequently thawed.

Saccharomyces cerevisiae. The test organism is grown overnight on culture medium Cm3 (pH 6.0–6.2 after sterilization) at a temperature of 35–37 °C. A suspension is prepared by washing off the growth with saline TS and diluting to a suitable opacity, for example, such that a 1-cm layer transmits 50 % of the incident light when examined at 650 nm. The suspension may be stored for up to 2 weeks at a temperature not exceeding 4 °C.

A freshly prepared inoculum may be replaced by a suitable suspension of the inoculum in a suitable vehicle, such as sterile peptone (1 g/l) TS2 that has been stored frozen at −70 °C and subsequently thawed.

Staphylococcus aureus. The test organism is grown overnight on culture medium Cm1 (pH 6.5–6.6 after sterilization) at a temperature of 35–37 °C. A suspension is prepared by washing off the growth with saline TS and diluting to a suitable opacity, for example, such that a 1-cm layer transmits 50 % of the incident light when examined at 650 nm.

A freshly prepared inoculum may be replaced by a suitable suspension of the inoculum in a suitable vehicle, such as sterile peptone (5 g/l) TS that has been stored frozen at −70 °C and subsequently thawed.

STERILITY TESTING OF ANTIBIOTICS

The test is designed to reveal the presence of contamination with live microorganisms in antibiotics intended for parenteral administration or for other sterile applications.

Test conditions

The test should be carried out under aseptic conditions in an area as free from contamination as it is possible to achieve by the use of disinfecting agents, germicidal lamps, and air filters. Germicidal lamps and disinfecting aerosols should not be used during actual testing operations. The test manipulations should be carried out in a filtered air environment or under a laminar flow hood, with operators dressed in sterilized, static-free clothing, including head and foot wear. The air pressure in the testing room should be greater than that of the exterior area. The performance of the laminar flow hood should be monitored by particulate count, settle plates, or slit-sampling devices, and the performance of the filters and germicidal lamps checked routinely.

Membrane filtration apparatus

A suitable unit consists of a closed reservoir and a receptacle, separated by a properly supported membrane of appropriate porosity. Membranes generally suitable for sterility testing have a nominal porosity of 0.45 μm, a diameter of approximately 47 mm, and a flow rate of 55–75 ml of water per minute at a pressure of 90 kPa (700 mm Hg). The entire unit should preferably be assembled and sterilized with the membrane in place, prior to use. If each entire membrane is to be cultured, at least 2 filter units should be set up.

All air entering the filtering unit should be passed through an air-filter capable of removing microorganisms.

Sampling

Take the sample in such a manner as to be representative of the material to be tested. The amount taken should be sufficient to perform the tests and any repeat tests that may be required. The sampling should be carried out in such a way as to maintain intact the sterility of the material.

Culture media

The culture media used for sterility tests for bacteria and fungi should be capable of supporting the growth of a wide variety of microorganisms, with both aerobic and anaerobic growth characteristics, including the types found in the environment of the manufacturing operations. More than one culture medium will generally be needed to fulfil these criteria. The media that usually give satisfactory results are fluid mercaptoacetate (thioglycolate) medium (culture medium Cm4) and soybean-casein digest medium (culture medium Cm5). Any other media that are used, however, should have at least demonstrably equivalent growth-supporting properties.

For testing the growth-supporting properties of each culture medium, strains of microorganisms should be used with exacting nutritive and aerobic-anaerobic requirements, in an inoculum containing only a small number of organisms (less than 100). The media should be incubated at the temperatures at which they will be used in the sterility test and growth should be evident after 24 hours.

Each lot of dehydrated medium obtained from a specialized manufacturer or each lot of the medium prepared entirely in the laboratory should be tested for its growth-supporting properties, since not every lot may support the growth of microorganisms to the desired extent. Differences may be caused by the occasional presence of unsatisfactory components in a particular lot, or by the destruction of certain components by overheating or oversterilization of the medium.

RECOMMENDED PROCEDURES

Membrane filtration test procedure

Aseptically transfer a suitable amount of the solid test material (0.3–6 g depending on the size of the container) into a sterile flask containing about 200 ml of peptone (1 g/l) TS1, stopper the flask and

swirl to effect rapid dissolution. If the test material dissolves slowly
or if the resulting solution will not filter rapidly, the volume of the solvent
may be increased to not more than 400 ml. Immediately after the test
material has dissolved, aseptically filter the solution, with the aid of
reduced pressure, through the membrane filter previously moistened
with sterile water or with peptone (1 g/l) TS1. To speed up the process
of filtration, the solution may be filtered using two filtering units simultaneously. To remove the residual antibiotic from the membrane, wash
it with sufficient peptone (1 g/l) TS1 to which, if so indicated in the
monograph (in the case of penicillin and cephalosporin antibiotics),
sufficient penicillinase TS has been added.

Upon completion of the filtration, divide the membrane aseptically
into two approximately equal parts. Transfer one part of the membrane
into a culture vessel (a test-tube is suitable) containing 50–100 ml of
culture medium Cm4 (fluid mercaptoacetate (thioglycolate) medium)
and the other part of the membrane into another culture vessel containing
50–100 ml of culture medium Cm5 (soybean-casein digest medium).

A control test should be carried out at appropriate intervals to
demonstrate that residual antibiotic activity is being reduced by the
above described washing procedure to below the level that allows growth
of an inoculum containing 50–100 microorganisms susceptible to the
antibiotic tested.

Direct test procedure

Depending on the size of the container take from 1–10 portions,
each 0.3 g of the test material, and aseptically transfer them into
individual sterile vessels (test-tubes are suitable) containing 50–100 ml
of culture medium Cm6 (fluid mercaptoacetate (thioglycolate) medium
with penicillinase). Transfer portions of similar size to another set of
individual sterile vessels containing 50–100 ml of culture medium Cm7
(soybean-casein digest medium with penicillinase).

Check the ability of the penicillinase contained in the medium to
inactivate all the penicillin in the test material by adding to one vessel
containing culture medium Cm6 the amount of material taken from
one container under test. Next add 1.0 ml of a dilution containing
50–100 microorganisms of a suitable strain (*Staphylococcus aureus*,
ATCC 6538-P is suitable) in culture medium Cm4. Typical microbial
growth must be observable after 24 hours of incubation at 30–32 °C.

Incubation

Incubate for 7 days the vessels containing fluid mercaptoacetate
(thioglycolate) media (culture media Cm4 and Cm6) at 30–32 °C and the
vessels containing soybean-casein digest media (media Cm5 and Cm7)

at 22–25 °C. In the direct test procedure, gently agitate the vessels at least once a day or until complete dissolution occurs.

If other culture media are used, the incubation temperature and the period of incubation may have to be appropriately modified.

Examine inoculated culture vessels at regular intervals and on the last day of incubation for evidence of microbial growth. If such growth is observed it should be confirmed by microscopic examination. It is desirable that the incubation apparatus be equipped with a continuous temperature-recording device.

Interpretation of test results

If no evidence of growth is found in any of the culture vessels, except in the positive growth control, the material meets the requirements of the test. If, however, evidence of growth is found, a repeat test may be performed. If no evidence of growth is then found in any of the culture vessels, except in the positive growth control, the material meets the requirement of the test. The material fails to pass the test if growth occurs in the repeat test.

The distinction between failure of the product to pass the test and a possible invalidity of the test procedure requires the competent judgement of an expert.

UNDUE TOXICITY

The test is used to determine the absence of undue toxicity of antibiotics intended for parenteral administration.

RECOMMENDED PROCEDURE

Use healthy mice of a single strain that have not previously been used for any test. Select 5 mice, each weighing between 18 g and 22 g. Prepare the solution of the test substance as specified in the monograph. Inject a test dose of 0.5 ml intravenously into a tail vein at a uniform rate, the injection occupying 5 seconds. Keep the mice under observation for 48 hours after the injection. The product meets the requirements for freedom from undue toxicity if no animal dies within 48 hours.

If 1 or 2 mice die within the observation period, repeat the procedure once, using respectively 5 or 15 mice, healthy and not previously used for any test, each weighing between 19.5 g and 20.5 g. The product under test meets the requirements for freedom from undue toxicity if no animal dies in the repeat test within the observation period (48 hours).

TEST FOR PYROGENS

The pyrogen test is designed to limit the risk of a febrile reaction following parenteral administration of drugs. It is intended to be used for liquid products that can be tolerated by the test rabbit in a dose of 10 ml per kg, injected intravenously, generally within a period of not more than 4 minutes. For products that require preliminary preparation or are subject to special conditions of administration, additional directions given in the monograph should be followed.

Test animal

Use healthy, adult rabbits, preferably of the same variety. House the animals individually in an area of uniform temperature (± 2 °C), possibly with uniform humidity, and free from disturbances likely to excite them. The animals are given *ad libitum* water and food, commonly used for laboratory animals. One to 3 days before using an animal that has not previously been used for a pyrogen test, condition it by conducting a training exercise as described under the recommended procedure, omitting the injection.

Do not use animals for pyrogen tests more frequently than once every 48 hours. After a pyrogen test in the course of which a rabbit's temperature has risen by 0.5 °C or more, or after a rabbit has been given a test substance that was adjudged pyrogenic, at least 2 weeks must be allowed to eapse before the animal is used again.

Temperature recording

Use an accurate thermometer graduated in 0.1 °C that has been tested to determine the time necessary to reach the maximum reading, or any other temperature-recording device of equal sensitivity. Insert the temperature-sensing device into the rectum of the test animal to a depth of about 6 cm. If the temperature-sensing device is to remain inserted throughout the sensing period, restrain the rabbit with a lightly-fitting neck stock that allows it to assume a natural resting posture. When a thermometer is used, allow sufficient time for it to reach a maximum temperature, as previously determined, before taking the reading.

RECOMMENDED PROCEDURE

Perform the test in the area where the animals are housed or under similar environmental conditions. For 2 hours before the test and during the test, withhold all food from the animals being used. Access to water may be allowed. The animals should be placed under the conditions of the test at least 1 hour before the injection.

Prior to the test, 40 minutes before the injection of the test material, determine the temperature of each animal by taking 2 measurements at an interval of 30 minutes. The mean of the 2 temperatures serves as the "control temperature" of the animal. The control temperature recorded for each rabbit constitutes the temperature from which any subsequent rise following the injection of the material is calculated.

In any one test, use only those animals the control temperatures of which do not deviate by more than 1.0 °C from each other. Those animals for which the 2 temperatures used to determine the control temperature have deviated by more than ± 0.2 °C from the mean should not be used in the test, nor should any animal with a control temperature below 38.0 °C or above 39.8 °C.

Render the syringes, needles, and glassware free from pyrogens by heating at 250 °C for not less than 30 minutes or by any other suitable method. Warm the solution to be tested to approximately 38 °C.

Inject into a marginal vein of the ear of each of 3 rabbits 10 ml of the solution per kg of body weight or the amount specified in the monograph. The injection should last not longer than 4 minutes, unless otherwise specified in the monograph.

When the injection has been completed, record the temperature of the animal during a period of 3 hours, taking the measurements continuously or every 30 minutes. The maximum temperature recorded for each rabbit is considered to be its response; if the temperature readings taken after the injection are all below the control temperature, the response is treated as a zero temperature rise.

If no rabbit shows an individual rise in temperature of 0.6 °C or more above its respective control temperature, and if the sum of the 3 temperature rises does not exceed 1.4 °C, the tested material meets the requirements for the absence of pyrogens. If 1 or 2 rabbits show a temperature rise of 0.6 °C or more, or if the sum of the temperature rises exceeds 1.4 °C, continue the test using 5 other rabbits. If not more than 3 of the 8 rabbits show individual rises in temperature of 0.6 °C or more, and if the sum of the 8 temperature rises does not exceed 3.7 °C, the tested material meets the requirements for the absence of pyrogens.

TEST FOR HISTAMINE-LIKE SUBSTANCES
(VASODEPRESSOR SUBSTANCES)

The test for vasodepressor substances is carried out in cats by comparing the depression of arterial pressure caused by the test solution with that obtained after administration of a solution of histamine.

RECOMMENDED PROCEDURES

Use healthy, adult cats, either males or non-pregnant females.

Determine the weight of the animal and place under general anaesthesia by injection of chloralose R or a suitable barbiturate that allows the maintenance of uniform blood pressure. Protect the animal from loss of body heat and maintain it so that the rectal temperature remains within physiological limits. Introduce a tube into the trachea. Surgically expose the common carotid artery and by blunt dissection separate it completely from all surrounding structures, including the vagus nerve. Insert a cannula filled with heparinized saline TS into the artery and connect it to a mercury manometer or another suitable device arranged for making a continuous record of blood pressure. Surgically expose the jugular or the femoral vein and insert into it another cannula filled with heparinized saline TS through which can be injected solutions of histamine and of the test substance.

Determine the sensitivity of the animal to histamine in the following way: Start the recording kymograph or a similar recording device and inspect the tracings for amplitude of excursion and relative stability of blood pressure. Inject into the jugular or femoral vein histamine TS, in doses of 0.05 µg (dose A), 0.1 µg (dose B) — repeated at least 3 times — and 0.15 µg (dose C) of histamine base per kg of animal weight. Administer the second and subsequent injections not less than 1 minute after the blood pressure has returned to the level recorded immediately before the previous injection. Repeat this series of injections until, disregarding the first series of readings, a relatively uniform decrease in blood pressure is obtained after doses B of histamine. The animal should be used for the test only if the decrease after doses B is not less than 2.7 kPa (20 mm Hg) and, moreover, if dose A causes smaller responses than doses B whereas dose C gives greater responses than doses B.

Prepare the test solution as described in the monograph. During the course of the test, take care to maintain a uniform rate of injection for both the test solution and the standard solution. If the jugular vein is used, care should also be taken that the injection of test solution and histamine standard are given in equal volumes to avoid volume effects on blood pressure. When a common cannula is used for both the standard and test solutions, each injection of the standard and test solution should be immediately followed by an injection of approximately 2.0 ml of saline TS to flush any residues from the tubing.

Inject a dose B of the standard solution followed by an injection of the specified amount of the test solution and then another dose B of the standard solution. The second and third injections are given not less than 1 minute after the blood pressure has returned to the level recorded immediately before the preceding injection. If the response to the test solution is greater than that given previously by dose A, repeat the series of injections twice and conclude the test by giving dose C of standard solution. If the response to dose C is not greater than that to dose B, the test is invalid.

The animal may be used in the test as long as it remains reasonably stable and responsive to histamine and provided that (*a*) an injection of test substance did not cause a greater depressor response than that caused by dose C and (*b*) the response to dose C of the standard solution given after the administration of the test substance does not become lower than the mean response to doses of B previously injected.

The substance passes the test if the response or the mean of the responses after the injection of the amount specified in the monograph is smaller than the mean of the corresponding responses to dose B of the standard solution (0.1 μg of histamine base per kg of animal weight), and no one single dose of the test solution causes a greater depressor response than dose C of the standard solution (0.15 μg of histamine base per kg of animal weight).

METHODS OF PHARMACOGNOSY

DETERMINATION OF ASH AND ACID-INSOLUBLE ASH

RECOMMENDED PROCEDURES

Determination of ash

Place about 3 g of the ground material, accurately weighed, or the quantity specified in the monograph, in a suitable tared dish (for example, of silica or platinum), previously ignited, cooled and weighed. Incinerate the material by gradually increasing the heat, not exceeding 450 °C, until free from carbon; cool, and weigh. If a carbon-free ash cannot be obtained in this way, exhaust the charred mass with hot water, collect the residue on an ashless filter-paper, incinerate the residue and filter-paper, add the filtrate, evaporate to dryness, and ignite at a temperature not exceeding 450 °C. Calculate the content in mg of ash per g of air-dried material.

Determination of acid-insoluble ash

Boil the ash for 5 minutes with 25 ml of hydrochloric acid ($\sim$70 g/l) TS; collect the insoluble matter in a sintered crucible, or on an ashless filter-paper, wash with hot water, and ignite at about 500 °C to constant weight. Calculate the content in mg of acid-insoluble ash per g of air-dried material.

MISCELLANEOUS

INTERNATIONAL CHEMICAL REFERENCE SUBSTANCES

A chemical reference substance is an authenticated uniform material that is intended for use in specified chemical, physical, and sometimes biological tests, in which its properties are compared with the properties of a product under examination; it possesses a degree of purity adequate for its intended use.

The types of analytical procedure at present used in specifications for pharmaceutical substances that may require a chemical reference substance are:

• infrared spectrophotometry, whether for identification or quantitative purposes;

• quantitative methods based on ultraviolet absorption spectrophotometry;

• quantitative methods based on the development of a colour and measurement of its intensity, whether by instrumental or visual comparison;

• methods based on chromatographic separation for identification or quantitative purposes;

• quantitative methods (including automated methods) based on other separative techniques that depend upon partition of the material to be determined between solvent phases, where the precise efficiency of the extraction procedure might depend upon ambient conditions that vary from time to time and from laboratory to laboratory;

• quantitative methods, often titrimetric but sometimes gravimetric, that are based on non-stoichiometric relationships;

• assay methods based on measurement of optical rotation;

• methods based on polarography;

• methods based on fluorescence spectrophotometry;

• microbiological assay methods based on the measurement of the inhibition of bacterial growth by antibiotics where the reference material may be adequately characterized by chemical and physical means (see "Microbiological assay of antibiotics", pp. 145-151).

A comprehensive discussion of the establishment, maintenance, and distribution of chemical reference substances is contained in Annex 3 to the twenty-fifth report of the WHO Expert Committee on Specifications for Pharmaceutical Preparations (WHO Technical Report Series, No. 567, 1975).

The International Chemical Reference Substances necessary to support the specifications of the *International Pharmacopoeia* are indicated in individual monographs of the pharmacopoeia.

International Chemical Reference Substances are established by the WHO Collaborating Centre for Chemical Reference Substances, Solna, Sweden. The characteristics of the substances selected are determined by the Centre in collaboration with specialists designated by WHO.

The International Chemical Reference Substances are available from the WHO Collaborating Centre for Chemical Reference Substances, Apotekens Centrallaboratorium, Box 3045, 171 03 Solna 3, Sweden. With each package of International Chemical Reference Substances there is included a leaflet giving analytical specifications for the substance and indicating the purpose for which it was established. On application to the Centre, additional information on analytical methodology will be supplied.

NAMES, SYMBOLS, AND RELATIVE ATOMIC MASSES OF CERTAIN ELEMENTS

The relative atomic mass (the term atomic weight was previously used) given in the table below is scaled relatively to the isotope ^{12}C taken as 12 exactly and is given to 4 significant figures. Only the elements most commonly encountered in pharmaceutical analysis are included.

Most elements have more than one naturally occurring isotope and the variation in the relative abundance of these isotopes influences the precision with which the relative atomic mass of an element in nature can be quoted. Among the elements included in the table, the relative atomic mass of samples in nature of boron, calcium, lead, strontium and sulfur may differ by more than one in the fourth significant figure.

Name	Symbol	Relative atomic mass	Name	Symbol	Relative atomic mass
Aluminium	Al	26.98	Cobalt	Co	58.93
Antimony	Sb	121.75*	Copper	Cu	63.55*
Arsenic	As	74.92	Fluorine	F	19.00
Barium	Ba	137.3	Gold	Au	197.0
Bismuth	Bi	209.0	Helium	He	4.003
Boron	B	10.81	Holmium	Ho	164.9
Bromine	Br	79.90	Hydrogen	H	1.008
Cadmium	Cd	112.4	Iodine	I	126.9
Calcium	Ca	40.08	Iron	Fe	55.85*
Carbon	C	12.01	Lanthanum	La	138.9
Cerium	Ce	140.1	Lead	Pb	207.2
Chlorine	Cl	35.45	Lithium	Li	6.941*
Chromium	Cr	52.00	Magnesium	Mg	24.31

* Values are considered reliable to ± 1 in the last digit or ± 3 when followed by an asterisk.

Name	Symbol	Relative atomic mass	Name	Symbol	Relative atomic mass
Manganese	Mn	54.94	Silver	Ag	107.9
Mercury	Hg	200.6*	Sodium	Na	22.99
Molybdenum	Mo	95.94	Strontium	Sr	87.62
Nickel	Ni	58.71*	Sulfur	S	32.06
Nitrogen	N	14.01	Thorium	Th	232.0
Oxygen	O	16.00*	Tin	Sn	118.7*
Phosphorus	P	30.97	Titanium	Ti	47.90*
Platinum	Pt	195.1*	Tungsten (Wolfram)	W	183.85*
Potassium	K	39.10*	Uranium	U	238.0
Ruthenium	Ru	101.1*	Vanadium	V	50.94*
Selenium	Se	78.96*	Zinc	Zn	65.38
Silicon	Si	28.09*	Zirconium	Zr	91.22

* Values are considered reliable to $\pm$ 1 in the last digit or $\pm$ 3 when followed by an asterisk.

LIST OF REAGENTS, TEST SOLUTIONS, AND VOLUMETRIC SOLUTIONS

The reagents, test solutions and volumetric solutions mentioned in the *International Pharmacopoeia*, 3rd edition, volume 1, are described below. The reagents are denoted by the abbreviation R, the test solutions by the abbreviation TS, and the volumetric solutions, or solutions that are similarly standardized, by the abbreviation VS. Similarly named reagents differing in composition, purity, etc., are distinguished by placing a numeral after the appropriate abbreviation. The designations AsR, AsTS, ClTS, FeTS and PbTS refer to reagents of suitable purity for use in the limit tests for arsenic, chlorides, iron, and heavy metals, respectively. The designation IR refers to reagents of suitable purity for use in spectrophotometry in the infrared region. The designation Cm denotes culture media for microbiological tests. The concentrations are expressed in conformity with the *Système international d'Unités* (SI) and they refer to the anhydrous substance. The reference to SRIP indicates *Specifications for reagents mentioned in the International Pharmacopoeia* (World Health Organization, Geneva, 1963). Designations previously used in SRIP are given in square brackets. The designation *d* denotes the relative density d_{20}^{20}, i.e., measured in air at 20 °C in relation to water at 20 °C.

Acetate buffer, pH 3.0, TS. A buffer mixture of pH 3.0.
Procedure. Dissolve 12 g of sodium acetate R in water, add 6 ml of glacial acetic acid R and dilute with sufficient water to produce 100 ml.

Acetic acid, glacial, R. $C_2H_4O_2$ (SRIP, 1963, p. 25); $d \sim 1.048$.

Acetic acid, glacial, R1. Glacial acetic acid R that complies with the following test: Mix 10.0 g with 10 ml of sulfuric acid ($\sim$1760 g/l) TS, cool to 20 °C, add 1 ml of potassium dichromate (0.0167 mol/l) VS, and allow to stand for 30 minutes. Add 50 ml of water, cool to 20 °C, add 1.5 ml of potassium iodide (80 g/l) TS, and titrate the liberated iodine with sodium thiosulfate (0.1 mol/l) VS, using starch TS as indicator. Not less than 0.6 ml of sodium thiosulfate (0.1 mol/l) VS is required.

Acetic acid ($\sim$300 g/l) TS. A solution of glacial acetic acid R containing about 300 g/l of $C_2H_4O_2$ (approximately 5 mol/l); $d \sim 1.037$.

Acetic acid ($\sim$60 g/l) TS. Acetic acid ($\sim$300 g/l) TS, diluted to contain about 60 g/l of $C_2H_4O_2$ (approximately 1 mol/l); $d \sim 1.008$.

Acetic acid ($\sim$60 g/l) PbTS. Acetic acid ($\sim$60 g/l) TS that complies with the following test: Evaporate 20 ml of acetic acid ($\sim$60 g/l) TS almost to dryness on a water-bath, add 25 ml of water and carry out the test for heavy metals. The heavy metals limit is 3 μg/ml.

Acetic anhydride R. $C_4H_6O_3$ (SRIP, 1963, p. 26).

Acetone R. C_3H_6O (SRIP, 1963, p. 27).

Acetonitrile R. Methyl cyanide, C_2H_3N.
Description. A clear, colourless liquid.
Miscibility. Freely miscible with water.

Acetonitrile (400 g/l) TS.
Procedure. Mix 1 volume of acetonitrile R with 1 volume of water. The resulting solution contains about 400 g/l of C_2H_3N.

Agar R. (SRIP, 1963, p. 27).

Aluminium hydroxide R. Hydrated $Al(OH)_3$.
Description. A white, odourless powder.
Solubility. Practically insoluble in water and in ethanol ($\sim$750 g/l) TS.

Ammonia ($\sim$260 g/l) TS [ammonia, strong, R]. (SRIP, 1963, p. 31); $d \sim 0.894$.

Ammonia ($\sim$100 g/l) TS. Ammonia ($\sim$260 g/l) TS, diluted to contain about 100 g/l of NH_3 (approximately 6 mol/l); $d \sim 0.956$.

Ammonia ($\sim$100 g/l) FeTS. Ammonia ($\sim$100 g/l) TS that complies with the following test: Evaporate 5 ml nearly to dryness on a water-bath, add 40 ml of water, 2 ml of citric acid (200 g/l) FeTS and 2 drops of thioglycolic acid R, mix, make alkaline with ammonia ($\sim$100 g/l) FeTS and dilute to 50 ml with water; no pink colour is produced.

Ammonia ($\sim$100 g/l) PbTS. Ammonia ($\sim$100 g/l) TS that complies with the following test: Evaporate 5 ml of ammonia ($\sim$100 g/l) TS to dryness on a water-bath, add to the residue 1 ml of hydrochloric acid ($\sim$70 g/l) TS, and evaporate to dryness. Dissolve the residue in 2 ml of acetic acid ($\sim$60 g/l) PbTS, dilute with water to 25 ml and carry out the test for heavy metals. Prepare the blank in a similar way. The heavy metals limit is 2 μg/ml.

Ammonia buffer TS.
Procedure. Dissolve 67.5 g of ammonium chloride R in 570 ml of ammonia ($\sim$260 g/l) TS and dilute with water to 1000 ml.

Ammonium acetate R. $C_2H_7NO_2$ (SRIP, 1963, p. 32).

Ammonium acetate (80 g/l) TS. A solution of ammonium acetate R containing about 77 g/l of $C_2H_7NO_2$ (approximately 1 mol/l).

Ammonium carbonate R. $(NH_4)_2CO_3$ (SRIP, 1963, p. 33).

Ammonium chloride R. NH_4Cl (SRIP, 1963, p. 33).

Ammonium chloride (10 μg/ml NH_4) TS.
Procedure. Dissolve 0.296 g, accurately weighed, of ammonium chloride R in sufficient water to produce 1000 ml. Dilute 10 ml of this solution to 100 ml.
Shelf-life. Use the solution within 2 weeks of its preparation.

Ammonium chloride buffer, pH 10.0, TS. A buffer mixture of pH 10.0.
Procedure. Dissolve 7.0 g of ammonium chloride R in 57 ml of ammonia ($\sim$260 g/l) TS and dilute with sufficient water to produce 100 ml.

Ammonium molybdate R. $(NH_4)_6Mo_7O_{24},4H_2O$ (SRIP, 1963, p. 34).

Ammonium molybdate (95 g/l) TS. A solution of ammonium molybdate R containing about 95 g/l of $(NH_4)_6Mo_7O_{24}$.

Ammonium oxalate R. $C_2H_8N_2O_4,H_2O$ (SRIP, 1963, p. 36).

Ammonium oxalate (25 g/l) TS. A solution of ammonium oxalate R containing about 27 g/l of $C_2H_8N_2O_4$.

Ammonium thiocyanate R. NH_4SCN (SRIP, 1963, p. 40).

Ammonium thiocyanate (75 g/l) TS. A solution of ammonium thiocyanate R containing about 75 g/l of NH_4SCN (approximately 1 mol/l).

Ammonium thiocyanate (0.1 mol/l) VS. Ammonium thiocyanate R, dissolved in water to contain 7.612 g of NH_4SCN in 1000 ml.
Method of standardization. Ascertain the exact concentration of the 0.1 mol/l solution in the following manner: Place 30.0 ml of silver nitrate (0.1 mol/l) VS in a glass-stoppered flask. Dilute with 50 ml of water, add 2 ml of nitric acid ($\sim$1000 g/l) TS and then titrate with the ammonium thiocyanate solution to the first appearance of a

red-brown colour, using 2 ml of ferric ammonium sulfate (45 g/l) TS as indicator.

Ammonium thiocyanate (0.01 mol/l) VS. Ammonium thiocyanate R, dissolved in water to contain 0.7612 g of NH_4SCN in 1000 ml.
Method of standardization. Ascertain the exact concentration of the solution following the method described under ammonium thiocyanate (0.1 mol/l) VS.

Antimony sodium tartrate R. $C_4H_4NaO_7Sb$.
Description. Hygroscopic, transparent or whitish scales or powder.
Solubility. Soluble in 1.5 parts of water; practically insoluble in ethanol ($\sim$710 g/l) TS.

Antimony sodium tartrate (50 g/l) TS. A solution of antimony sodium tartrate R containing about 50 g/l of $C_4H_4NaO_7Sb$.

Arsenic, dilute, AsTS. One millilitre contains 10 μg of arsenic.
Procedure. Dilute 1 ml of strong arsenic AsTS with sufficient water to produce 100 ml.
Note: Dilute arsenic AsTS must be freshly prepared.

Arsenic, strong, AsTS.
Procedure. Dissolve 0.132 g of arsenic trioxide R in 6 ml of sodium hydroxide ($\sim$80 g/l) TS, by gentle heating. Dilute the cooled solution with 20 ml of water, and add 50 ml of hydrochloric acid ($\sim$250 g/l) TS and sufficient water to produce 100 ml.

Arsenic trioxide R. As_2O_3 (SRIP, 1963, p. 44).

Barium chloride R. $BaCl_2,2H_2O$ (SRIP, 1963, p. 45).

Barium chloride (50 g/l) TS. A solution of barium chloride R containing about 52 g/l of $BaCl_2$ (approximately 0.25 mol/l).

Barium chloride (0.5 mol/l) VS. Barium chloride R, dissolved in water to contain 104.2 g of $BaCl_2$ in 1000 ml.
Method of standardization. Ascertain the exact concentration of the 0.5 mol/l solution in the following manner: Place 10.0 ml of sulfuric acid (0.5 mol/l) VS in a flask, dilute with 40 ml of water, add 2 drops of thorin (2 g/l) TS and titrate slowly with the barium chloride solution to a reddish colour.

Barium nitrate R. $Ba(NO_3)_2$ (SRIP, 1963, p. 47).

Barium nitrate (0.01 mol/l) VS. Barium nitrate R, dissolved in water to contain 2.614 g of $Ba(NO_3)_2$ in 1000 ml.
Method of standardization. Ascertain the exact concentration of the 0.01 mol/l solution in the following manner: Place 10.0 ml of sulfuric acid (0.01 mol/l) VS in a flask, dilute with 40 ml of water, add 2 drops of thorin (2 g/l) TS and 2 drops of methylthioninium chloride (0.2 g/l) TS, and titrate slowly with the barium nitrate solution from yellow to a pink colour.

Barium oxide R. BaO.
Description. White to yellowish-white lumps or powder. Absorbs moisture and carbon dioxide on exposure to air.
Storage. Store in tightly closed containers.

Barium sulfate suspension TS.
Procedure. Mix 15 ml of barium chloride (0.5 mol/l) VS with 55 ml of water and 20 ml of sulfate-free ethanol (~750 g/l) TS, add 5 ml of potassium sulfate (174 mg/l) TS, and dilute with sufficient water to produce 100 ml.
Note. Barium sulfate suspension TS must be freshly prepared.

Beef extract R. A residue from beef broth obtained by extracting fresh, sound, lean beef by cooking with water and evaporating the resulting broth at a low temperature, usually under reduced pressure until a thick pasty residue is obtained.

Benzylpenicillin sodium R. $C_{16}H_{17}N_2NaO_4S$. Contains not less than 96.0 % and not more than 102.0 % of $C_{16}H_{17}N_2NaO_4S$, calculated with reference to the dried substance.
Description. A white or almost white, crystalline powder; odourless or with a faint characteristic odour.
Solubility. Soluble in about 0.5 part of water; practically insoluble in chloroform R and ether R.

Benzylpenicillin sodium TS.
Procedure. Dissolve 0.03 g of benzylpenicillin sodium R in sufficient phosphate buffer, pH 7.0, TS, to produce 10 ml. This solution contains not less than 3 mg/ml of benzylpenicillin sodium R.

Boric acid R. H_3BO_3. Contains not less than 99.0 % of H_3BO_3.
Description. White crystals or scales of a somewhat pearly lustre or a white, crystalline powder.
Solubility. Soluble in 20 parts of water, in 3 parts of boiling water, and in 16 parts of ethanol (~750 g/l) TS.
Water-insoluble substances. 1.0 g dissolves in 30 parts of water; the solution is clear and colourless.
Ethanol-insoluble substances. 1.0 g dissolves in 10 ml of boiling ethanol (~750 g/l) TS; the solution is not more than faintly turbid.
Assay. Dissolve about 1 g, accurately weighed, in 30 ml of water; add 50 ml of glycerol R, previously neutralized to phenolphthalein/ethanol TS, and titrate with carbonate-free sodium hydroxide (1 mol/l) VS, using phenolphthalein/ethanol TS as indicator. Each ml of carbonate-free sodium hydroxide (1 mol/l) VS is equivalent to 61.83 mg of H_3BO_3.

Boric acid (50 g/l) TS. A solution of boric acid R containing about 50 g/l of H_3BO_3.

Bromine R. Br_2 (SRIP, 1963, p. 51).

Bromine TS1. A saturated solution of bromine R.

Bromine AsTS.

Procedure. Dissolve 30 g of potassium bromide R in 40 ml of water, add 30 g of bromine R and dilute with sufficient water to produce 100 ml. The solution complies with the following test: Evaporate 10 ml nearly to dryness on a water-bath, add 50 ml of water, 10 ml of hydrochloric acid ($\sim$250 g/l) AsTS, and sufficient stannous chloride AsTS to reduce the remaining bromine, and apply the general test for arsenic. The colour of the stain produced is not more intense than that produced from a 1-ml standard stain, showing that the amount of arsenic does not exceed 1μ g/ml.

Bromophenol blue R. $C_{19}H_{10}Br_4O_5S$ (SRIP, 1963, p. 52).

Bromophenol blue/ethanol TS.

Procedure. Warm 0.1 g of bromophenol blue R with 3.2 ml of sodium hydroxide (0.05 mol/l) VS and 5 ml of ethanol ($\sim$710 g/l) TS; after solution has been effected, add a sufficient quantity of ethanol ($\sim$150 g/l) TS to produce 250 ml.

Bromothymol blue R. $C_{27}H_{28}Br_2O_5S$ (SRIP, 1963, p. 53).

Bromothymol blue/ethanol TS.

Procedure. Warm 0.1 g of bromothymol blue R with 3.2 ml of sodium hydroxide (0.05 mol/l) VS and 5 ml of ethanol ($\sim$710 g/l) TS; after solution has been effected, add a sufficient quantity of ethanol ($\sim$150 g/l) TS to produce 250 ml.

Brown stock standard TS.

Procedure. To 35.0 ml of cobalt colour TS, add 17.0 ml of copper colour TS, 8.0 ml of dichromate colour TS, dilute to 100.0 ml with iron colour TS, and mix.

Calcium carbonate R1. $CaCO_3$ (SRIP, 1963, p. 56).

Calcium carbonate R2. $CaCO_3$. Calcium carbonate R1 of suitable quality to serve as a primary standard for the standardization of disodium edetate.

Calcium chloride, anhydrous, R [calcium chloride R]. $CaCl_2$ (SRIP, 1963, p. 58).

Calcium chloride, hydrated, R. $CaCl_2,6H_2O$ (SRIP, 1963, p. 58).

Calcium chloride (55 g/l) TS. A solution of hydrated calcium chloride R containing about 55 g/l of $CaCl_2$ (approximately 0.5 mol/l).

Calcon R. Monosodium salt of 2-hydroxy-1-[(2-hydroxy-1-naphthyl)-azo]naphthalene-4-sulfonic acid; C.I. Mordant Black 17, C.I. No. 15705, Eriochrome Blue Black R, Solochrome Dark Blue; $C_{20}H_{13}N_2NaO_5S$.

Calcon carboxylic acid R. 2-Hydroxy-1-(2-hydroxy-4-sulfo-1-naphthylazo)-3-naphthoic acid; $C_{21}H_{14}N_2O_7S,3H_2O$.
Description. A dark-brown powder with a violet tint.
Solubility. Practically insoluble in water; slightly soluble in methanol R and in ethanol ($\sim$750 g/l) TS; freely soluble in solutions of alkali hydroxides.

Calcon carboxylic acid indicator mixture R.
Procedure. Mix 0.1 g of calcon carboxylic acid R with 10 g of anhydrous sodium sulfate R.

Calcon indicator mixture R.
Procedure. Mix 0.1 g of calcon R with 10 g of anhydrous sodium sulfate R.

Carbon dioxide R. CO_2.
Description. A colourless gas; odourless.
Solubility. Soluble in about 1.3 parts by volume of water.

Carbon disulfide R. CS_2 (SRIP, 1963, p. 62).

Carbon disulfide IR. Carbon disulfide R that complies with the following test: The infrared absorption spectrum of a 1.0-mm layer, as described in method 4 under "Spectrophotometry in the infrared region" (see p. 42), and examined over the range 4000–670 cm^{-1} shows an absorbance of less than 0.1 in the regions 4000–3030 cm^{-1}, 2635–2440 cm^{-1}, 2000–1755 cm^{-1}, and 1265–935 cm^{-1}, and an absorbance of less than 0.17 in the region 800–715 cm^{-1}.

Carbon tetrachloride R. CCl_4 (SRIP, 1963, p. 63).

Ceric ammonium nitrate R. $Ce(NO_3)_4,2NH_4NO_3$.
Description. Small orange-red monoclinic crystals.
Solubility. Very soluble in water.
Insoluble matter. To 5 g, accurately weighed, add 10 ml of sulfuric acid ($\sim$1760 g/l) TS, stir, and cautiously add 90 ml of water to dissolve. Heat to boiling and digest in a covered beaker on a water-bath for 1 hour. Filter through a tared filtering crucible, wash thoroughly, and dry at 105 °C. The weight of the residue does not exceed 2.5 mg.
Assay. Dissolve 2.5 g, accurately weighed and previously dried at 85 °C for 24 hours, in 10 ml of sulfuric acid ($\sim$190 g/l) TS and add 40 ml of water. Add a few drops of *o*-phenanthroline TS and titrate with ferrous sulfate (0.1 mol/l) VS. Each ml of ferrous sulfate (0.1 mol/l) VS is equivalent to 54.8 mg of $Ce(NO_3)_4, 2 NH_4NO_3$.

Ceric ammonium nitrate TS.
Procedure. Dissolve 6.25 g of ceric ammonium nitrate R in 10 ml of nitric acid (15 g/l) TS.
Shelf-life. Use within 3 days of preparation.

Ceric sulfate R. Usually $Ce(SO_4)_2,4H_2O$ (SRIP, 1963, p. 63).

Ceric sulfate (35 g/l) TS. A solution of ceric sulfate R containing about 33 g/l of $Ce(SO_4)_2$.

Charcoal R. (SRIP, 1963, p. 64).

Chloralose R. $C_8H_{11}Cl_3O_6$.
Description. A colourless, crystalline powder.
Melting temperature. About 187 °C.
Specific optical rotation. Use a 50 mg/ml solution in ethanol ($\sim$750 g/l) TS; $[\alpha]_D^{20\,°C} = + 19°$.

Chlorine R. Cl_2 (SRIP, 1963, p. 65).

Chlorine TS. A saturated solution of chlorine R in water.
Note: Chlorine TS must be freshly prepared.

Chloroform R. $CHCl_3$ (SRIP, 1963, p. 66).

Citric acid R. $C_6H_8O_7,H_2O$ (SRIP, 1963, p. 69).

Citric acid FeR. Citric acid R that complies with the following test: Dissolve 0.5 g of citric acid R in 40 ml of water, add 2 drops of mercaptoacetic acid R, mix, make alkaline with ammonia ($\sim$100 g/l) FeTS and dilute to 50 ml with water; no pink colour is produced.

Citric acid (180 g/l) FeTS. A solution of citric acid FeR containing about 183 g/l of $C_6H_8O_7$.

Cobalt colour, strong, TS.
Procedure. Dissolve 8.0 g of cobaltous chloride R in 120 ml of sulfuric acid ($\sim$10 g/l) TS, filter the solution, if necessary, and determine the concentration of $CoCl_2,6H_2O$.
Assay. Dilute 5.0 ml with sufficient water to produce 100 ml. Transfer 10.0 ml of this solution to a glass-stoppered flask, add 10 ml of water, 0.5 ml of hydrogen peroxide ($\sim$60 g/l) TS and 10 ml of sodium hydroxide ($\sim$80 g/l) TS. Add a few boiling chips to the flask, and boil the contents of the flask until the excess of hydrogen peroxide is completely decomposed (approximately 10 minutes). Cool the flask, add 20 ml of water, 1 g of potassium iodide R, and 25 ml of hydrochloric acid (2 mol/l) VS. Close the flask with the stopper and allow to stand until the precipitate dissolves. Titrate the liberated iodine with sodium thiosulfate (0.01 mol/l) VS using starch TS as indicator. Each ml of sodium thiosulfate (0.01 mol/l) VS is equivalent to 2.380 mg of $CoCl_2,6H_2O$.

Cobalt colour TS. A solution containing 60.0 g/l of $CoCl_2,6H_2O$.
Procedure. Prepare a solution containing 6.000 g of $CoCl_2,6H_2O$ in 100 ml by diluting the strong cobalt colour TS with sulfuric acid ($\sim$10 g/l) TS, as necessary.

Cobaltous chloride R. $CoCl_2,6H_2O$ (SRIP, 1963, p. 70).

Congo red paper R. (SRIP, 1963, p. 72).

Copper colour, strong, TS.

Procedure. Dissolve 8.0 g of copper(II) sulfate R in 120 ml of sulfuric acid ($\sim$10 g/l) TS, filter the solution, if necessary, and determine the concentration of $CuSO_4,5H_2O$.

Assay. Dilute 5.0 ml with sufficient water to produce 100 ml. Transfer 10.0 ml of this solution to a glass-stoppered flask, add 20 ml of water, 1 g of potassium iodide R, and 5 ml of glacial acetic acid R. After 10 minutes, titrate the liberated iodine with sodium thiosulfate (0.01 mol/l) VS, using starch TS as indicator. Each ml of sodium thiosulfate (0.01 mol/l) VS is equivalent to 2.497 mg of $CuSO_4,5H_2O$.

Copper colour TS. A solution containing 60.0 g/l of $CuSO_4,5H_2O$.

Procedure. Prepare a solution containing 6.000 g of $CuSO_4,5H_2O$ in 100 ml by diluting the strong copper colour TS with sulfuric acid ($\sim$10 g/l) TS, as necessary.

Copper(II) sulfate R. $CuSO_4,5H_2O$ (SRIP, 1963, p. 72).

Copper(II) sulfate (160 g/l) TS. A solution of copper(II) sulfate R containing about 160 g/l of $CuSO_4$.

Crystal violet R. $C_{25}H_{30}ClN_3$ (SRIP, 1963, p. 73).

Crystal violet/acetic acid TS. A solution of crystal violet R dissolved in glacial acetic acid R1 containing about 5 g/l.

Culture medium Cm1.

Procedure. Dissolve 6.0 g of dried peptone R, 4.0 g of pancreatic digest of casein R, 3.0 g of water-soluble yeast extract R, 1.5 g of beef extract R, 1.0 g of glucose hydrate R, and 10–20 g of agar R in sufficient water to produce 1000 ml.

Note: The quantity of agar R used should permit the culture medium to be of adequate firmness to support cylinders or to permit holes to be cut without tearing the gel layer.

Culture medium Cm2.

Procedure. Dissolve 17.0 g of pancreatic digest of casein R, 3.0 g of papaic digest of soybean meal R, 5.0 g of sodium chloride R, 2.5 g of dipotassium hydrogen phosphate R, 2.5 g of glucose hydrate R, and 10–20 g of agar R in about 500 ml of water. Heat the solution, add 10.0 g of polysorbate 80 R and dilute immediately with a sufficient amount of water to produce 1000 ml.

Note: The quantity of agar R used should permit the culture medium to be of adequate firmness to support cylinders or to permit holes to be cut without tearing the gel layer.

Culture medium Cm3.

Procedure. Dissolve 9.4 g of dried peptone R, 4.7 g of water-soluble yeast extract R, 2.4 g of beef extract R, 10.0 g of sodium chloride R,

10.0 g of glucose hydrate R, and 15–25 g of agar R in sufficient water to produce 1000 ml.

Note: The quantity of agar R used should permit the culture medium to be of adequate firmness to support cylinders or to permit holes to be cut without tearing the gel layer.

Culture medium Cm4. Fluid mercaptoacetate (thioglycolate) medium. *Procedure.* Thoroughly grind in a mortar in the following order: 0.5 g of L-cystine R, 2.5 g of sodium chloride R, 5.5 g of glucose hydrate R, 0.75 g of agar R, 5.0 g of water-soluble yeast extract R and 15.0 g of pancreatic digest of casein R. Add a small volume of hot water, transfer to a suitable container, and add sufficient water to produce 1000 ml. Complete the solution by heating in a boiling water-bath, taking care to ensure complete solution of the L-cystine R. Add 0.3 ml of mercaptoacetic acid R or 0.5 g of sodium mercaptoacetate R (the latter is preferred as a more stable compound) and sufficient sodium hydroxide (1 mol/l) VS so that the pH of the final and sterilized medium will be 7.0–7.2. Reheat the solution, but do not boil, filter, if necessary, through cotton wool and add 1.0 ml of resazurin sodium (1 g/l) TS. Distribute the solution into suitable vessels and sterilize by autoclaving for 18–20 minutes at 121 °C and cool promptly to 25 °C. *Storage.* At 20–30 °C, avoiding excessive light.

Note: If the uppermost portion of the medium has changed to a pink colour and this exceeds one-fifth of the depth of the medium, it is unsuitable for use, but may be restored once by heating in steam.

Culture medium Cm5. Soybean-casein digest medium. *Procedure.* Dissolve in water 17.0 g of pancreatic digest of case in R, 3.0 g of papaic digest of soybean meal R, 5.0 g of sodium chloride R, 2.5 g of dipotassium hydrogen phosphate R, and 2.5 g of glucose hydrate R. Warm the solution slightly, then cool it to room temperature and add sufficient water to produce 1000 ml. Adjust the pH of the solution with sodium hydroxide (1 mol/l) VS, if necessary, so that the pH of the final and sterilized medium will be 7.1–7.5. Filter, if necessary to clarify, distribute the solution into suitable vessels and sterilize in an autoclave for 18–20 minutes at 121 °C.

Culture medium Cm6. Fluid mercaptoacetate (thioglycolate) medium with penicillinase. *Procedure.* Use culture medium Cm4 with sufficient sterile penicillinase TS added to inactivate the penicillin activity of the test material. Add penicillinase TS to individual vessels containing sterile culture medium Cm4 using an aseptic technique. Prior to use, or at the time of the test, incubate a representative number of the vessels with culture medium Cm6 at 30–32 °C for 24–48 hours and examine for sterility.

Culture medium Cm7. Soybean-casein digest medium with penicillinase.
Procedure. Use culture medium Cm5 to which 5.0 ml of polysorbate 80 R has been added before sterilization and with sufficient sterile penicillinase TS added to inactivate the penicillin activity of the test material. Add penicillinase TS to individual vessels containing sterile culture medium Cm5, using an aseptic technique.

Cyclohexane R. C_6H_{12} (SRIP, 1963, p. 74).

L-Cystine R. $C_6H_{12}N_2O_4S_2$ (SRIP, 1963, p. 75).

Dibromomethane R. Methylene bromide, CH_2Br_2.
Description. Colourless to yellowish liquid.
Miscibility. Miscible with ethanol (~750 g/l) TS, ether R, and acetone R.

Dichloromethane R. Methylene chloride, CH_2Cl_2.
Description. A clear colourless, mobile liquid.
Miscibility. Freely miscible with ethanol (~750 g/l) TS and ether R.
Boiling range. Not less than 95 % distils between 39 and 41 °C.
Residue on evaporation. Leaves, after evaporation on a water-bath and drying at 105 °C, not more than 0.5 mg/ml.

Dichromate colour, strong, TS.
Procedure. Dissolve 6.0 g of potassium dichromate R in 120 ml of sulfuric acid (~10 g/l) TS, filter the solution, if necessary, and determine the concentration of $K_2Cr_2O_7$.
Assay. Dilute 5.0 ml with sufficient water to produce 50 ml. Transfer 10.0 ml of this solution to a glass-stoppered flask, add 10 ml of water, 2 g of potassium bicarbonate R, and 20 ml of sulfuric acid (~100 g/l) TS. Loosely close the flask with its stopper. When the gas evolution has ceased, add 1 g of potassium iodide R, keep the flask for 5 minutes in a dark place and titrate the liberated iodine with sodium thiosulfate (0.1 mol/l) VS, using starch TS as indicator. Each ml of sodium thiosulfate (0.1 mol/l) VS is equivalent to 4.904 mg of $K_2Cr_2O_7$.

Dichromate colour TS. A solution containing 4.904 g/l of $K_2Cr_2O_7$.
Procedure. Prepare a solution containing 490.35 mg of $K_2Cr_2O_7$ in 100 ml by diluting the strong dichromate colour TS with sulfuric acid (~10 g/l) TS, as necessary.

Diethylene glycol R. $C_4H_{10}O_3$.
Description. A colourless to faintly yellow liquid having a mild odour.
Miscibility. Freely miscible with water, ethanol (~750 g/l) TS, ether R and acetone R.
Boiling range. Between 240 and 250 °C.

Mass density (ϱ_{20}). 1.117–1.120 kg/l.

Acidity. Transfer 60 g to a 250-ml conical flask, add phenolphthalein/ethanol TS and titrate with potassium hydroxide/ethanol (0.02 mol/l) VS, to a pink colour that remains stable for at least 15 seconds. Not more than 2.5 ml should be consumed.

Dimethylformamide R. C_3H_7NO.

Description. A clear and colourless liquid, having a characteristic odour.

Miscibility. Miscible with water and ethanol ($\sim$750 g/l) TS.

Boiling range. Not less than 25 % distils at between 152 and 156 °C.

Mass density (ϱ_{20}). 0.945–0.947 kg/l.

Acidity and alkalinity. Dissolve 1 g in 10 ml of water, add 2 drops of phenolphthalein/ethanol TS; not more than 0.2 ml of carbonate-free sodium hydroxide (0.01 mol/l) VS is required to produce a red colour. Add 0.3 ml of hydrochloric acid (0.01 mol/l) VS and 5 drops of methyl.red/ethanol TS; an orange colour is produced.

1,4-Di[2-(4-methyl-5-phenyloxazole)]benzene R.   Dimethyl-POPOP

$C_{26}H_{20}N_2O_2$. Suitable for scintillation counting.

Dioxan R.   1,4-Dioxane, $C_4H_8O_2$.

Caution. It is dangerous to determine the boiling range or the residue on evaporation before complying with the test for peroxides.

Description. A clear, colourless liquid.

Miscibility. Miscible with water, ethanol ($\sim$750 g/l) TS and ether R.

Boiling range. Not less than 95 % distils at between 101 and 105 °C.

Melting temperature. Solidifies when cooled in ice and does not completely remelt at temperatures below 10 °C.

Residue on evaporation. Evaporate on a water-bath and dry to constant weight at 105 °C; it leaves a residue of not more than 0.1 mg/ml.

Mass density (ϱ_{20}). About 1.031 kg/l.

Water. Determined by the Karl Fischer method, not more than 5.0 mg/ml.

Peroxide. Add 5 ml to a mixture of 1 g of potassium iodide R dissolved in 10 ml of water, 5 ml of hydrochloric acid ($\sim$70 g/l) TS, and 2 ml of starch TS, and mix; not more than a faint blue or brown colour is produced.

Diphenylbenzidine R. $C_{24}H_{20}N_2$.

Description. A white, or faintly grey-coloured, crystalline powder.

Solubility. Insoluble in water; slightly soluble in ethanol ($\sim$750 g/l) TS and acetone R.

Melting range. 246–250 °C.

Sulfated ash. Not more than 1.0 mg/g.

Nitrates. Dissolve 8 mg in a cooled mixture of nitrogen-free sulfuric acid ($\sim$1760 g/l) TS and 5 ml of water; the solution is colourless or not more than very pale blue.

Diphenylcarbazone R. $C_{13}H_{12}N_4O$ (SRIP, 1963, p. 81).

Diphenylcarbazone/ethanol TS. A solution of diphenylcarbazone R dissolved in ethanol ($\sim$750 g/l) TS containing about 1 g/l of $C_{13}H_{12}N_4O$.

Diphenyl ether R. Phenyl ether, $C_{12}H_{10}O$.
Description. A colourless liquid.
Miscibility. Immiscible with water; freely miscible with glacial acetic acid R and with most organic solvents.
Boiling temperature. About 259 °C.
Melting range. 26–28 °C.

2,5-Diphenyloxazole R. PPO, $C_{15}H_{11}NO$. Suitable for scintillation counting.

Dipotassium hydrogen phosphate R. K_2HPO_4 (SRIP, 1963, p. 81).

Disodium edetate R. $C_{10}H_{14}N_2Na_2O_8,2H_2O$ (SRIP, 1963, p. 82).

Disodium edetate (0.05 mol/l) VS. Disodium edetate R, dissolved in water to contain 16.81 g of $C_{10}H_{14}N_2Na_2O_8$ in 1000 ml.
Method of standardization. Ascertain the exact concentration by an appropriate method. The following method is suitable: Transfer about 200 mg of calcium carbonate R2, accurately weighed, to a 400-ml beaker, add 10 ml of water, and swirl to form a slurry. Cover the beaker with a watch glass, and introduce 2 ml of hydrochloric acid ($\sim$70 g/l) TS from a pipette inserted between the lip of the beaker and the edge of the watch glass. Swirl the contents of the beaker to dissolve the calcium carbonate. Wash down the sides of the beaker, the outer surface of the pipette, and the watch glass with water, and dilute with water to about 100 ml. While stirring the solution, preferably with a magnetic stirrer, add about 30 ml of the disodium edetate solution from a 50-ml burette. Add 10 ml of sodium hydroxide ($\sim$80 g/l) TS and 0.3 g of calcon indicator mixture R or of calcon carboxylic acid indicator mixture R and continue the titration with the disodium edetate solution to a blue end-point. Each 5.005 mg of calcium carbonate is equivalent to 1 ml of disodium edetate (0.05 mol/l) VS.

Disodium hydrogen phosphate, anhydrous, R [sodium phosphate, anhydrous, R]. Na_2HPO_4 (SRIP, 1963, p. 193).

Ethanol, dehydrated, R. C_2H_5OH (SRIP, 1963, p. 85).

Ethanol ($\sim$750 g/l) TS [ethanol (95 per cent) R] (SRIP, 1963, p. 84).

Ethanol ($\sim$750 g/l), sulfate-free, TS. Ethanol ($\sim$750 g/l) TS that complies with the following test: Evaporate 25 ml of ethanol ($\sim$750 g/l) TS to a volume of about 2 ml, add a mixture of 3 ml of hydrochloric acid ($\sim$70 g/l) TS and 42 ml of water, and 5 ml of barium sulfate suspension TS. Proceed as described in "Limit test for sulfates" (see p. 116). Sulfate-free ethanol ($\sim$750 g/l) TS contains not more than 20 µg/ml.

Ethanol ($\sim$710 g/l) TS. A solution of about 950 ml of ethanol ($\sim$750 g/l) TS diluted with water to 1000 ml.

Ethanol ($\sim$375 g/l) TS. A solution of about 525 ml of ethanol ($\sim$750 g/l) TS diluted with water to 1000 ml.

Ethanol ($\sim$150 g/l) TS. A solution of about 210 ml of ethanol ($\sim$750 g/l) TS diluted with water to 1000 ml.

Ether R. $C_4H_{10}O$ (SRIP, 1963, p. 85).

Ethyl acetate R. $C_4H_8O_2$ (SRIP, 1963, p. 86).

Ethylene glycol monoethyl ether R. $C_4H_{10}O_2$.
Description. A clear, colourless liquid.
Miscibility. Miscible with water, ethanol ($\sim$750 g/l) TS, ether R, and acetone R.
Boiling range. Not less than 95 % distils at between 133 and 135 °C.
Mass density (ϱ_{20}). About 0.93 kg/l.

Ferric ammonium sulfate R. $FeNH_4(SO_4)_2,12H_2O$ (SRIP, 1963, p. 88).

Ferric ammonium sulfate (45 g/l) TS. A solution of ferric ammonium sulfate R containing about 45 g/l of $FeNH_4(SO_4)_2$.

Ferric chloride R. $FeCl_3,6H_2O$ (SRIP, 1963, p. 88).

Ferric chloride (25 g/l) TS. A solution of ferric chloride R containing about 27 g/l of $FeCl_3$.

Ferrous ammonium sulfate R. $Fe(NH_4)_2(SO_4)_2,6H_2O$ (SRIP, 1963, p. 89).

Ferrous ammonium sulfate (1 g/l) TS. A solution of ferrous ammonium sulfate R containing about 1 g/l of $Fe(NH_4)_2(SO_4)_2$.

Ferrous sulfate R. $FeSO_4,7H_2O$ (SRIP, 1963, p. 90).

Ferrous sulfate (15 g/l) TS. A solution of ferrous sulfate R in freshly boiled and cooled water containing about 15 g/l of $FeSO_4$ (approximately 0.1 mol/l).
Note: Ferrous sulfate (15 g/l) TS must be freshly prepared.

Ferrous sulfate (0.1 mol/l) VS.
Procedure. Dissolve 2.8 g of ferrous sulfate R in 90 ml of freshly boiled and cooled water, and add a sufficient quantity of sulfuric acid ($\sim$1760 g/l) TS to produce 100 ml.

Method of standardization. Ascertain the exact concentration of the 0.1 mol/l solution in the following manner: To 40.0 ml of the ferrous sulfate solution add 5 ml of phosphoric acid ($\sim$1,440 g/l) TS and titrate immediately with potassium permanganate (0.02 mol/l) VS. *Note:* Standardize immediately before use.

Formic acid ($\sim$1080 g/l) TS [formic acid R]. CH_2O_2 (SRIP, 1963, p. 92) *d* $\sim$1.2.

Gelatin R. Gelatin of suitable purity.

Gelatin TS. A solution of gelatin R dissolved in phosphate buffer, pH 7.0, TS containing about 10 g/l.

Glucose hydrate R. Monohydrate of α-D-glucopyranose, $C_6H_{12}O_6$, H_2O. Contains not less than 99.0 % and not more than 101.5 % of $C_6H_{12}O_6$, calculated with reference to the dried substance.
Description. Colourless crystals or a white crystalline or granular powder; odourless.
Solubility. Soluble in about 1 part of water and in about 60 parts of ethanol ($\sim$750 g/l) TS; more soluble in boiling water and in boiling ethanol ($\sim$750 g/l) TS.
Acidity. Dissolve 5 g in 50 ml of carbon-dioxide-free water R. It requires for neutralization not more than 0.5 ml of carbonate-free sodium hydroxide (0.02 mol/l) VS, phenolphthalein/ethanol TS being used as indicator.
Specific optical rotation. Dissolve 100 mg, previously dried to constant weight, in 1 ml of water, and add a few drops of ammonia ($\sim$100 g/l) TS; $[\alpha]_D^{20\,°C} = + 52$ to $+ 53°$.
Soluble starch or sulfites. Dissolve 1 g in 10 ml of water and add 1 drop of iodine TS; the liquid is coloured yellow.
Loss on drying. Dry to constant weight at 105 °C; it loses not less than 80 mg/g and not more than 100 mg/g.
Sulfated ash. Not more than 1.0 mg/g.
Assay. Dissolve about 0.1 g, accurately weighed, in 50 ml of water, add 30 ml of iodine (0.1 mol/l) VS, 10 ml of sodium carbonate (50 g/l) TS, and allow to stand for 20 minutes. Add 15 ml of hydrochloric acid ($\sim$70 g/l) TS and titrate the excess of iodine with sodium thiosulfate (0.1 mol/l) VS, using starch TS as indicator. Perform a blank determination and make any necessary corrections. Each ml of iodine (0.1 mol/l) VS is equivalent to 9.008 mg of $C_6H_{12}O_6$.

Glycerol R. Propane-1,2,3-triol with small amounts of water, $C_3H_8O_3$. Contains not less than 970 g/kg of $C_3H_8O_3$.
Description. A clear, almost colourless, syrupy and hygroscopic liquid; odourless.

Miscibility. Miscible with water and ethanol ($\sim$750 g/l) TS; practically immiscible with ether R and chloroform R.

Mass density (ϱ_{20}). Not less than 1.256 kg/l.

Refractive index (n_D^{20}). Not less than 1.469.

Acrolein and other reducing substances. Mix 1 ml with 1 ml of ammonia ($\sim$100 g/l) TS and heat in a water-bath at 60 °C for 5 minutes; the liquid is not coloured yellow. Remove from the water-bath and add 3 drops of silver nitrate (40 g/l) TS; the liquid does not become coloured within 5 minutes.

Sulfated ash. Not more than 0.5 mg/ml.

Glyoxal bis(2-hydroxyanil) R. 2,2′-(Ethanediylidenedinitrilo)diphenol, $C_{14}H_{12}N_2O_2$.

Description. White crystals.

Solubility. Soluble in hot ethanol ($\sim$750 g/l) TS.

Melting temperature. 203–205 °C.

Glyoxal bis(2-hydroxyanil) TS. A solution of glyoxal bis(2-hydroxyanil) R dissolved in ethanol ($\sim$750 g/l) TS containing about 10 g/l of $C_{14}H_{12}N_2O_2$.

Green stock standard TS.

Procedure. To 3.5 ml of cobalt colour TS, add 20.1 ml of copper colour TS, 10.4 ml of dichromate colour TS, and 4.0 ml of iron colour TS; dilute to 100.0 ml with sulfuric acid ($\sim$10 g/l) TS, and mix.

Helium R. He. Contains not less than 999.95 ml/l of He.

Heparinized saline TS. A sterile solution of saline TS containing 50 International Units of heparin in 1 ml.

Histamine, strong, TS. A solution containing 1.00 g/l of histamine base.

Procedure. Dissolve 138.1 mg, accurately weighed, of histamine phosphate R or 82.8 mg, accurately weighed, of histamine dihydrochloride R in sufficient water to produce 50.0 ml.

Storage. Strong histamine TS should be stored at a temperature not exceeding 4–10 °C, in dark glass bottles with ground-glass stoppers, protected from light.

Shelf-life. Do not use longer than 30 days.

Histamine TS. A solution containing 1.0 mg/l of histamine base.

Procedure. Prepare histamine TS by diluting strong histamine TS with a sufficient quantity of saline TS.

Note: Histamine TS must be freshly prepared.

Histamine dihydrochloride R. $C_5H_9N_3,2HCl$. Contains not less than 98.0 %, and not more than 101.0 % of $C_5H_9N_3,2HCl$, calculated with reference to the dried substance.

Description. Colourless crystals or a white crystalline powder; odourless.

Solubility. Freely soluble in water and in methanol R; soluble in ethanol ($\sim$750 g/l) TS.

Melting range. 244–246 °C.

Loss on drying. Not more than 5.0 mg/g.

Assay. Dissolve about 0.15 g, accurately weighed, in 10 ml of water. Add 5 ml of chloroform R and 25 ml of ethanol ($\sim$750 g/l) TS. Titrate with carbonate-free sodium hydroxide (0.2 mol/l) VS, using 0.5 ml of thymolphthalein/ethanol TS as indicator. Each ml of carbonate-free sodium hydroxide (0.2 mol/l) VS is equivalent to 9.21 mg of $C_5H_9N_3,2HCl$.

Histamine phosphate R. $C_5H_9N_3,2H_3PO_4$. Contains not less than 98.0 %, and not more than 101.0 % of $C_5H_9N_3,2H_3PO_4$, calculated with reference to the anhydrous substance.

Description. Colourless, long, prismatic crystals; odourless. Stable in air.

Solubility. Soluble in about 5 parts of water; slightly soluble in ethanol ($\sim$750 g/l) TS.

Melting temperature. About 132 °C.

Water. Determined by the Karl Fischer method, using about 1.0 g, the water content is 50–60 mg/g.

Assay. Dissolve about 0.15 g, accurately weighed, in 10 ml of water. Add 5 ml of chloroform R and 25 ml of ethanol ($\sim$750 g/l) TS. Titrate with carbonate-free sodium hydroxide (0.2 mol/l) VS, using 0.5 ml of thymolphthalein/ethanol TS as indicator. Each ml of carbonate-free sodium hydroxide (0.2 mol/l) VS is equivalent to 15.36 mg of $C_5H_9N_3,2H_3PO_4$.

Holmium oxide R. Ho_2O_3. Contains not less than 99.9 % of Ho_2O_3, the impurities consisting of Er_2O_3 and Dy_2O_3.

Description. A tan-coloured powder.

Solubility. Insoluble in water.

Holmium perchlorate TS.

Procedure. Dissolve 40 g of holmium oxide R in sufficient perchloric acid ($\sim$140 g/l) TS to produce 1000 ml.

Hydriodic acid ($\sim$970 g/l) TS [hydriodic acid R]. HI (SRIP, 1963, p. 95).

Hydrochloric acid ($\sim$420 g/l) TS [hydrochloric acid, saturated, R]. (SRIP, 1963, p. 96); $d \sim 1.18$.

Hydrochloric acid ($\sim$250 g/l) TS. A solution of hydrochloric acid ($\sim$420 g/l) TS in water, containing approximately 250 g/l of HCl; $d \sim 1.12$.

Hydrochloric acid ($\sim$250 g/l) AsTS. Hydrochloric acid ($\sim$250 g/l) TS that complies with the following tests A and B:

A. Dilute 10 ml with sufficient water to produce 50 ml, add 5 ml of ammonium thiocyanate (75 g/l) TS and stir immediately; no colour is produced.

B. To 50 ml add 0.2 ml of bromine AsTS, evaporate in a water-bath until reduced to 16 ml, adding more bromine AsTS if necessary to ensure that an excess, as indicated by the colour, is present throughout the evaporation. Add 50 ml of water and 5 drops of stannous chloride AsTS and apply the general test for arsenic. The colour of the stain produced is not more intense than that produced from a 0.2-ml standard stain, showing that the amount of arsenic does not exceed 0.05 µg/ml.

Hydrochloric acid (~250 g/l), stannated, AsTS.
Procedure. Dilute 1 ml of stannous chloride AsTS with sufficient hydrochloric acid (~250 g/l) AsTS to produce 100 ml.

Hydrochloric acid (~70 g/l) TS.
Procedure. Dilute 260 ml of hydrochloric acid (~250 g/l) TS with sufficient water to produce 1000 ml (approximately 2 mol/l); $d \sim 1.035$.

Hydrochloric acid ClTS. One millilitre contains 50 µg of Cl.
Procedure. Dilute 14.3 ml of hydrochloric acid (0.1 mol/l) VS with sufficient water to produce 1000 ml.

Hydrochloric acid (2 mol/l) VS. Hydrochloric acid (~250 g/l) TS, diluted with water to contain 72.93 g of HCl in 1000 ml.
Method of standardization. Ascertain the exact concentration of the solution following the method described under hydrochloric acid (1 mol/l) VS.

Hydrochloric acid (1 mol/l) VS. Hydrochloric acid (~250 g/l) TS, diluted with water to contain 36.47 g of HCl in 1000 ml.
Method of standardization. Ascertain the exact concentration of the 1 mol/l solution in the following manner: Dissolve about 1.5 g, accurately weighed, of anhydrous sodium carbonate R, previously dried at 270 °C for 1 hour, in 50 ml of water and titrate with the hydrochloric acid solution, using methyl orange/ethanol TS as indicator. Each 52.99 mg of anhydrous sodium carbonate is equivalent to 1 ml of hydrochloric acid (1 mol/l) VS.

Hydrochloric acid (0.5 mol/l) VS. Hydrochloric acid (~250 g/l) TS, diluted with water to contain 18.23 g of HCl in 1000 ml.
Method of standardization. Ascertain the exact concentration of the solution following the method described under hydrochloric acid (1 mol/l) VS.

Hydrochloric acid (0.1 mol/l) VS. Hydrochloric acid (~250 g/l) TS, diluted with water to contain 3.647 g of HCl in 1000 ml.
Method of standardization. Ascertain the exact concentration of the solution following the method described under hydrochloric acid (1 mol/l) VS.

Hydrochloric acid (0.015 mol/l) VS. Hydrochloric acid ($\sim$250 g/l) TS, diluted with water to contain 0.5470 g of HCl in 1000 ml.
Method of standardization. Ascertain the exact concentration of the solution following the method described under hydrochloric acid (1 mol/l) VS.

Hydrochloric acid (0.01 mol/l) VS. Hydrochloric acid ($\sim$250 g/l) TS, diluted with water to contain 0.3647 g of HCl in 1000 ml.
Method of standardization. Ascertain the exact concentration of the solution following the method described under hydrochloric acid (1 mol/l) VS.

Hydrogen peroxide ($\sim$60 g/l) TS. A solution in water containing about 60 g of H_2O_2 per litre.

Hydrogen sulfide R. H_2S (SRIP, 1963, p. 98).

Hydrogen sulfide TS. A saturated solution of hydrogen sulfide R in cold water.
Note: Hydrogen sulfide TS must be freshly prepared.

Iodine R. I_2 (SRIP, 1963, p. 101).

Iodine TS.
Procedure. Dissolve 2.6 g of iodine R and 3 g of potassium iodide R in sufficient water to produce 100 ml (approximately 0.2 mol/l).

Iodine (0.1 mol/l) VS. Iodine R and potassium iodide R, dissolved in water to contain 12.69 g of I and 18.0 g of KI in 1000 ml.
Method of standardization. Ascertain the exact concentration of the 0.1 mol/l solution by titrating 25.0 ml with sodium thiosulfate (0.1 mol/l) VS, using starch TS as indicator.

Iodine (0.02 mol/l) VS. Iodine R and potassium iodide R, dissolved in water to contain 2.538 g of I and 3.6 g of KI in 1000 ml.
Method of standardization. Ascertain the exact concentration of the solution following the method described under iodine (0.1 mol/l) VS.

Iodine (0.01 mol/l) VS. Iodine R and potassium iodide R, dissolved in water to contain 1.269 g of I and 3.6 g of KI in 1000 ml.
Method of standardization. Ascertain the exact concentration of the solution following the method described under iodine (0.1 mol/l) VS.

Iodine bromide R. IBr.
Description. Blue-black or brownish-black crystals.
Solubility. Freely soluble in water, ethanol ($\sim$750 g/l) TS, chloroform R, ether R, and glacial acetic acid R.
Melting temperature. About 40 °C.
Storage. Store in a cool place, in a tightly closed container, protected from light.

Iodine bromide TS.

Procedure. Dissolve 20 g of iodine bromide R in sufficient glacial acetic acid R to produce 1000 ml.

Storage. Store in a tightly closed container, protected from light.

Iron colour, strong, TS.

Procedure. Dissolve 6.6 g of ferric chloride R in 120 ml of sulfuric acid ($\sim$10 g/l) TS, filter the solution, if necessary, and determine the concentration of $FeCl_3,6H_2O$.

Assay. Dilute 5.0 ml with sufficient water to produce 25.0 ml. Transfer 10.0 ml of this solution to a flask, and add 60 ml of water. Adjust the pH to 2–3 with hydrochloric acid (1 mol/l) VS and ammonia ($\sim$100 g/l) TS, using congo red paper R. Heat the solution to approximately 45 °C, and titrate with disodium edetate (0.05 mol/l) VS, using 2 ml of sulfosalicylic acid (175 g/l) TS as indicator, until the solution changes from a lilac tint to straw-yellow. Each ml of disodium edetate (0.05 mol/l) VS is equivalent to 13.52 mg of $FeCl_3,6H_2O$.

Iron colour TS. A solution containing 45.0 mg/ml of $FeCl_3,6H_2O$.

Procedure. Prepare a solution containing 4.500 g of $FeCl_3,6H_2O$ in 100 ml, diluting the strong iron colour TS with sulfuric acid ($\sim$10 g/l) TS, as necessary.

Iron standard FeTS.

Procedure. Dissolve 0.173 g of ferric ammonium sulfate R in 100 ml of water, add 5 ml of hydrochloric acid ($\sim$70 g/l) TS and sufficient water to produce 1000 ml. Each ml of this solution contains 20 μg of iron.

Karl Fischer reagent TS. A freshly prepared solution contains up to 5.0 mg/ml of water. The solution should not be used if the water equivalent falls below 2.5 mg of water per ml of the reagent.

Procedure. Dissolve 63 g of iodine R in 100 ml of anhydrous pyridine R, cool in ice, and pass sulfur dioxide R into the solution until a gain in weight of 32 g has occurred, taking care to avoid absorption of atmospheric moisture. Add sufficient dehydrated methanol R to produce 500 ml and allow to stand for 24 hours. Karl Fischer reagent TS may also be prepared by mixing commercially available solutions of sulfur dioxide in pyridine and of iodine in methanol, which are stable when properly stored, for example, protected from light. The resulting solution should conform to the requirements stated below.

Method of standardization. Ascertain the exact content of water in the following manner: Add about 20 ml of dehydrated methanol R, to the titration vessel and titrate to the endpoint with Karl Fischer reagent TS without recording the volume required. Introduce in an appropriate form a suitable amount of water, accurately weighed, and titrate again to the endpoint with Karl Fischer reagent TS, recording the volume. Water might be introduced, for example, as a solution in dry methanol, or under the form of a hydrated compound. Calculate the water equivalent of the reagent in mg of water per ml. Karl Fischer reagent TS deteriorates continuously and should be standardized immediately before use, or daily, as required.

Note: Ethylene glycol monoethyl ether R may be used in the preparation of the reagent instead of dehydrated methanol R.

Lanthanum nitrate R. $La(NO_3)_3,6H_2O$. Contains not less than 97.0 % of $La(NO_3)_3$, $6 H_2O$.

Description. Colourless crystals; deliquescent.

Solubility. Freely soluble in water.

Assay. Dissolve about 0.75 g, accurately weighed, in 25 ml of water, add 3 ml of nitric acid ($\sim$130 g/l) TS, 3 g of methenamine R, and about 20 mg of xylenol orange indicator mixture R, and titrate with disodium edetate (0.05 mol/l) VS until the solution becomes pure yellow in colour. If fading of the colour of the indicator occurs towards the end of the titration, more methenamine R should be added. Each ml of disodium edetate (0.05 mol/l) VS is equivalent to 21.65 mg of $La(NO_3)_3,6H_2O$.

Lanthanum nitrate (30 g/l) TS.

Procedure. Dissolve 4.3 g of lanthanum nitrate R in 1 ml of nitric acid ($\sim$130 g/l) TS and sufficient water to produce 100 ml.

Lead, strong, PbTS. One millilitre contains 100 μg of lead.

Procedure. Dissolve 0.1598 g of lead nitrate R in 5 ml of nitric acid ($\sim$1000 g/l) TS and sufficient water to produce 1000 ml.

Lead, dilute, PbTS. One millilitre contains 10 μg of lead.

Procedure. Dilute 10 ml of strong lead PbTS with sufficient water to produce 100 ml.

Note: Dilute lead PbTS must be freshly prepared.

Lead acetate R. $C_4H_6O_4Pb$, $3 H_2O$ (SRIP, 1963, p. 105).

Lead acetate (80 g/l) TS. A solution of lead acetate R in freshly boiled water containing about 80 g/l of $C_4H_6O_4Pb$ (approximately 0.25 mol/l).

Lead nitrate R. $Pb(NO_3)_2$ (SRIP, 1963, p. 107).

Lead nitrate (0.05 mol/l) VS. Lead nitrate R, dissolved in water to contain 16.56 g of $Pb(NO_3)_2$ in 1000 ml.

Method of standardization. Ascertain the exact concentration of the 0.05 mol/l solution by diluting 25.0 ml with 200 ml of water, add 10 ml of ammonia buffer TS and about 20 mg of Mordant Black 11 indicator mixture R, and titrate with disodium edetate (0.05 mol/l) VS.

Lithium perchlorate R. $LiClO_4$.

Description.   Small crystals.

Solubility.   Freely soluble in water; sparingly soluble in ethanol ($\sim$750 g/l) TS, acetone R, ether R, and ethyl acetate R.

Lithium perchlorate/acetic acid TS.

Procedure.   Dissolve 10.64 g of lithium perchlorate R in sufficient glacial acetic acid R1 to produce 1000 ml.

Macrogol 400 R.   Polyethylene glycol 400.   Macrogol 400 R is a polymer of ethylene oxide and water, represented by the formula $H(OCH_2CH_2)_nOH$, in which the average value of n lies between 8.2 and 9.1.

Description.   Clear colourless (or practically colourless) viscous liquid having a slight characteristic odour; slightly hygroscopic.

Average molecular weight.   Transfer to a pressure flask 2.1 g of macrogol 400 R, accurately weighed, and 25.0 ml of phthalic anhydride/ pyridine TS.   Insert the stopper in the flask, wrap the flask securely with cloth, and immerse it in a water-bath maintained at 96–100 °C, to the same depth as the mixture in the flask, for 1 hour.   Remove the flask, retaining the cloth wrapping, and allow to cool in air to room temperature.   To the contents of the flask add 50 ml of carbonate-free sodium hydroxide (0.5 mol/l) VS and 5 drops of phenolphthalein/ pyridine TS.   Titrate with carbonate-free sodium hydroxide (0.5 mol/l) VS to a pink endpoint that remains for not less than 15 seconds.   Perform a blank determination in a similar manner.   Calculate the average molecular weight by multiplying by 4000 the weight, in g, of the test substance and dividing the result by the difference between the volume, in ml, of carbonate-free sodium hydroxide (0.5 mol/l) VS consumed for the test substance and the blank determination.   The average molecular weight is between 380 and 420.

Mass density (ϱ_{20}).   1.110–1.140 kg/l.

Congealing point.   Between 4 and 8 °C, the congealing point being the average of 4 consecutive temperature readings, the highest and lowest of which differ by not more than 0.4 °C.

pH Value.   Between 4.5 and 7.5, in a 50 g/l solution.

Acidity or alkalinity.   Dissolve 5.0 g in 50 ml of water.   Add a few drops of phenol red/ethanol TS.   If the solution turns yellow, titrate with sodium hydroxide (0.01 mol/l) VS; if the solution turns red, titrate with hydrochloric acid (0.01 mol/l) VS.   Not more than 2.0 ml of titrant should be required in either case.

Sulfated ash.   Not more than 10 mg/g.

Heavy metals.   Mix 4 g, accurately weighed, with 1 ml of hydrochloric acid ($\sim$70 g/l) TS and dilute with water to 25 ml.   The limit is 50 μg/g.

Limit of monoethylene and diethylene glycols.   Dissolve 50 g in 75 ml of diphenyl ether R in a 250-ml distillation flask. Slowly distil at a pressure of 100-250 Pa (1–2 mmHg) into a receiver that is graduated to 100 ml in 1-ml subdivisions, until 25 ml of distillate have been collected. Add 25.0 ml of water to the distillate, shake the receiving flask vigorously, and allow the layers to separate. Cool the container in an ice-bath to solidify and facilitate the removal of the layer of diphenyl ether R. Filter the water layer through filter-paper into a glass-stoppered, 50-ml graduated cylinder. To the filtrate add an equal volume of freshly distilled acetonitrile R, and shake the cylinder until solution is complete. Pipette 10 ml of the solution into 15 ml of ceric ammonium nitrate TS, mix, and within 2–5 minutes determine the absorbance of the resulting solution at about 525 nm. Use a blank consisting of 15 ml of ceric ammonium nitrate TS and 10 ml of acetonitrile (400 g/l) TS. Prepare a standard solution by mixing 10 ml of acetronile (400 g/l) TS, to which 30 mg of diethylene glycol R have been added, and 15 ml of ceric ammonium nitrate TS and determine the absorbance within 2-5 minutes at about 525 nm, using the same blank as above. The absorbance of the test solution should not exceed that of the standard solution.

Magnesium oxide R. MgO.
Description. A white, very fine powder.
Solubility. Very slightly soluble in water; insoluble in ethanol ($\sim$750 g/l) TS.

Magnesium sulfate R. $MgSO_4, 7H_2O$ (SRIP, 1963, p. 111).

Manganese dioxide R. MnO_2 (SRIP, 1963, p. 112).

Manganese/silver paper R.
Procedure. To a mixture of equal volumes of silver nitrate (0.1 mol/l) VS and manganese sulfate (15 g/l) TS, add drop by drop sodium hydroxide (0.1 mol/l) VS until a persistent precipitate is produced, and filter. Soak strips of filter-paper (Whatman No. 1 is suitable) for 15 minutes in the solution, dry them at ambient temperature, protected from light and acidic or alkaline vapours. The manganese/silver paper R should be colourless.
Test for sensitivity. Place in a cylinder of about 40 ml capacity (height about 80 mm, internal diameter about 30 mm) 1.0 ml of ammonium chloride (10 μg/ml NH_4) TS. Add 9 ml of water and 1 g of magnesium oxide R. Immediately stopper the flask using a polyethylene cap below which a manganese/silver paper R is placed. Swirl the solution carefully so that magnesium particles do not come into contact with the reagent paper. Keep the cylinder at 50–60 °C for 1 hour. A true grey colour is produced on the reagent paper.

Manganese sulfate R. $MnSO_4,H_2O$.
Description. Pale-red, slightly efflorescent crystals.
Solubility. Soluble in about 1 part of water and 0.6 part of boiling water; practically insoluble in ethanol ($\sim$750 g/l) TS.

Manganese sulfate (15 g/l) TS. Manganese sulfate R, dissolved in water to contain 15.0 g/l of $MnSO_4$.

Mercaptoacetic acid R (thioglycolic acid R). $C_2H_4O_2S$ (SRIP, 1963, p. 206).

Mercuric acetate R. $C_4H_6HgO_4$ (SRIP, 1963, p. 112).

Mercuric acetate/acetic acid TS.
Procedure. Dissolve 50 g of mercuric acetate R in sufficient glacial acetic acid R1, that has been neutralized, if necessary, to crystal violet/acetic acid TS with perchloric acid (0.1 mol/l) VS, to produce 1000 ml.

Mercuric bromide R. $HgBr_2$ (SRIP, 1963, p. 113).

Mercuric bromide AsTS.
Procedure. Dissolve 5 g of mercuric bromide R in sufficient ethanol ($\sim$750 g/l) TS to produce 100 ml.

Mercuric bromide paper AsR.
Procedure. Use smooth, white filter-paper weighing 65–120 g/m². The thickness of the paper in mm should be approximately equal numerically to the weight expressed as above, divided by 400. Soak pieces of filter-paper, not less than 25 mm in width, in mercuric bromide AsTS, decant the superfluous liquid, suspend the paper over a non-metallic thread, and allow it to dry, protected from light.
Storage. Store the mercuric bromide paper AsR in stoppered bottles in the dark.
Note: Paper that has been exposed to sunlight or to vapours of ammonia must not be used as it produces only a pale stain or no stain at all.

Mercuric nitrate R. $Hg(NO_3)_2,H_2O$.
Caution. Mercuric nitrate R is poisonous.
Description. A white or slightly yellow, deliquescent, crystalline powder.
Solubility. Soluble in water in the presence of a small quantity of nitric acid ($\sim$1000 g/l) TS.

Mercuric nitrate (0.01 mol/l) VS.
Procedure. Dissolve about 3.5 g, accurately weighed, of mercuric nitrate R in a mixture of 5 ml of nitric acid ($\sim$1000 g/l) TS and 500 ml of water, and dilute with water to 1000 ml.
Method of standardization. Ascertain the exact concentration of the 0.01 mol/l solution in the following manner: Transfer 20.0 ml to a conical flask, add 2 ml of nitric acid ($\sim$1000 g/l)TS and 2 ml of

ferric ammonium sulfate (45 g/l) TS. Cool to below 20 °C, and titrate with ammonium thiocyanate (0.01 mol/l) VS to the first appearance of a permanent brownish colour.

Mercuric oxide, yellow, R. HgO (SRIP, 1963, p. 114).

Mercuric sulfate TS.
Procedure. Mix 5 g of yellow mercuric oxide R with 40 ml of water and, while stirring, add 20 ml of sulfuric acid (~1760 g/l) TS, then add 40 ml of water and stir until completely dissolved.

Methanol, dehydrated, R. Methanol R that complies with the following requirement: Water, not more than 1.0 mg/g.

Methanol R. CH_3OH (SRIP, 1963, p. 117).

Methenamine R. Hexamethylenetetramine, $C_6H_{12}N_4$. Contains not less than 99.0 % of $C_6H_{12}N_4$.
Description. Colourless crystals or a crystalline powder; odourless.
Solubility. Soluble in water and ethanol (~750 g/l) TS.
Acidity and alkalinity. Dissolve 2.5 g in 25 ml of water. To 10 ml add 3 drops of phenolphthalein/ethanol TS; a pink colour is produced, which changes to red after the addition of 1 drop of carbonate-free sodium hydroxide (0.1 mol/l) VS. To a further 10 ml aliquot add 3 drops of bromothymol blue/ethanol TS; a blue colour is produced, which changes to green-blue after the addition of 3 drops of hydrochloric acid (0.1 mol/l) VS.
Sulfated ash. Not more than 0.5 mg/g.
Assay. Dissolve about 1.5 g, accurately weighed, in 10 ml of water, add 50 ml of sulfuric acid (0.5 mol/l) VS, and boil until the odour of formaldehyde is no longer perceptible. Titrate the excess of acid with sodium hydroxide (1 mol/l) VS, using methyl red/ethanol TS as indicator. Each ml of sulfuric acid (0.5 mol/l) VS is equivalent to 35.05 mg of $C_6H_{12}N_4$.

Methyl orange R. Sodium salt of 4'-dimethylaminoazobenzene-4-sulfonic acid, $C_{14}H_{14}N_3NaO_3S$ (SRIP, 1963, p. 118).

Methyl orange/ethanol TS.
Procedure. Dissolve 0.04 g of methyl orange R in sufficient ethanol (~150 g/l) TS to produce 100 ml.

Methyl red R. 4'-Dimethylaminoazobenzene-2-carboxylic acid, $C_{15}H_{15}N_3O_2$ (SRIP, 1963, p. 118).

Methyl red/ethanol TS.
Procedure. Dissolve 25 mg of methyl red R in a mixture of 0.95 ml of sodium hydroxide (0.05 mol/l) VS and 5 ml of ethanol (~750 g/l) TS, warm the solution slightly and after cooling dilute with sufficient ethanol (~375 g/l) TS to produce 250 ml.

Methyl red/methylthioninium chloride TS.
Procedure. Mix 20 ml of a 0.5 mg/ml solution of methyl red R in ethanol (∼150 g/l) TS with 0.4 ml of a 20 mg/ml solution of methylthioninium chloride R in water.

Methylthioninium chloride R [methylene blue]. $C_{16}H_{18}ClN_3S,3H_2O$ (SRIP, 1963, p. 119).

Methylthioninium chloride (0.2 g/l) TS.
Procedure. Dissolve 23 mg of methylthioninium chloride R in sufficient water to produce 100 ml.

Mordant Black 11 R [eriochrome black R]. C.I. Mordant Black 11, C.I. No. 14645, Eriochrome Black T, Solochrome Black; sodium salt of 2-(2-hydroxy-6-nitro-4-sulfo-1-naphthylazo)-1-naphthol, $C_{20}H_{12}N_3NaO_7S$ (SRIP, 1963, p. 84).

Mordant Black 11 indicator mixture R.
Procedure. Mix 1 g of Mordant Black 11 R with 100 g of sodium chloride R.

2-Naphthol R [β-naphthol R]. $C_{10}H_8O$ (SRIP, 1963, p. 122).

2-Naphthol TS1.
Procedure. Dissolve 5 g of 2-naphthol R, freshly recrystallized, in 40 ml of sodium hydroxide (∼80 g/l) TS and add sufficient water to produce 100 ml.
Note: 2-Naphthol TS1 must be freshly prepared.

Nitric acid (∼1000 g/l) TS [nitric acid (70 per cent.) R]. (SRIP, 1963, p. 125); $d \sim 1.41$.

Nitric acid (∼130 g/l) TS.
Procedure. Dilute 130 ml of nitric acid (∼1000 g/l) TS with sufficient water to produce 1000 ml (approximately 2 mol/l); $d \sim 1.07$.

Nitric acid (15 g/l) TS. Nitric acid (∼1000 g/l) TS, diluted with water to contain 15.0 g/l of HNO_3.

Nitric acid (3 g/l) TS. Nitric acid (∼1000 g/l) TS, diluted with water to contain 3.0 g/l of HNO_3.

Nitrobenzene R. $C_6H_5NO_2$ (SRIP, 1963, p. 128).

Nitrogen R. N_2 (SRIP, 1963, p. 129).

Pancreatic digest of casein R. (SRIP, 1963, p. 132).

Papaic digest of soybean meal R. (SRIP, 1963, p. 134).

Paraffin, liquid, R. (SRIP, 1963, p. 135).

Penicillinase R. An enzyme, usually obtained from culture filtrates of a strain of *Bacillus cereus*, which has the specific property of inactivating penicillin by splitting the bond linking the nitrogen of the thiazolidine

to the adjacent carbonyl carbon and thus releasing a carboxyl group. It is precipitated from solutions in water by acetone R, ethanol ($\sim$750 g/l) TS, and dioxan R, but inactivated by several hours' contact with these solvents; it is rapidly inactivated by ethyl acetate R. In place of penicillinase R a sterile filtrate obtained by fermentation of a penicillinase-producing organism in a suitable medium, described below under "Preparation of penicillinase", may also be used directly.
Description. Small, brown, easily pulverizable pieces or granules.
Solubility. Freely soluble in water, forming a slightly opalescent solution.

Preparation of penicillinase. Dissolve 10 g of pancreatic digest of casein R, 2.7 g of potassium dihydrogen phosphate R, and 5.9 g of sodium citrate R in 200 ml of water, adjust the alkalinity to pH 7.2 with sodium hydroxide ($\sim$200 g/l) TS, and dilute to 1000 ml with water. Dissolve 0.4 g of magnesium sulfate R in 5 ml of water and add 1 ml of ferrous ammonium sulfate (1 g/l) TS and sufficient water to produce 10 ml. Sterilize both solutions by heating in an autoclave, cool, mix, distribute in shallow layers in conical flasks and inoculate with a suitable strain (*Bacillus cereus*, NCTC 9946, is suitable). Allow the flasks to stand at 18-37 °C until growth is apparent and then maintain at 35-37 °C for 16 hours, shaking constantly to ensure maximum aeration. Centrifuge and sterilize the supernatant liquid by filtration through a suitable membrane filter.

Penicillinase TS. A sterile aqueous solution of penicillinase R.
To test the activity of penicillinase TS, carry out the "Penicillinase assay". The time required for iodine decolorization is not more than 36 seconds.

Penicillinase assay. Carry out the assay in test-tubes of borosilicate glass, 15 cm long and about 20 mm in internal diameter, immersed in a water-bath of 30 ± 1 °C. All reagents should have a temperature of 30 °C before use.
To the test-tube add the reagents in the following order: 1.6 ml of gelatin TS. 0.4 ml of penicillinase TS to be tested, 1 drop of starch TS, and 1 ml of benzylpenicillin sodium TS, blowing out the last reagent from a 1-ml pipette. Start the stop-watch and after 15 seconds add 2.0 ml of iodine (0.01 mol/l) VS, recording the time of decolorization of iodine from the time of the addition of benzylpenicillin sodium TS. The activity of penicillinase TS is calculated from the results of the assay. The time of decolorization of strictly 36 seconds corresponds to a penicillinase activity equivalent to a rate of decomposition (at 30 °C at pH 7.0) of 220 mg of benzylpenicillin sodium R per hour per ml of penicillinase TS.
Storage. Store between 0 and 2 °C and use within 2–3 days. When

dried from the frozen state and kept in sealed ampoules, penicillinase TS may be stored for several months.

Peptone, dried, R. (SRIP, 1963, p. 137).

Peptone R1. Dried peptone R that conforms to the following requirement: An autoclaved solution containing 0.02 g/ml is clear and neutral or almost neutral.

Peptone (5 g/l) TS.
Procedure. Dissolve in water, while heating, 5.0 g of dried peptone R and 7 g of sodium chloride R and dilute with sufficient water to produce 1000 ml. Adjust to pH 8.0–8.4 and boil for 20 minutes. Filter, adjust to pH 7.2–7.4, and sterilize by maintaining at 115 °C for 30 minutes.

Peptone (1 g/l) TS1.
Procedure. Dissolve 1.0 g of peptone R1 (or similar peptic digest of animal tissue) in sufficient water to produce 1000 ml, filter or centrifuge to clarify, adjust the pH to 7.1 ± 0.2, place 100 ml portions into individual vessels, and sterilize by maintaining at 121 °C for 18–20 minutes.

Peptone (1 g/l) TS2.
Procedure. Dissolve in water, while heating, 1.0 g of dried peptone R and 9 g of sodium chloride R and dilute with sufficient water to produce 1000 ml. Adjust to pH 8.0–8.4 and boil for 20 minutes. Filter, adjust to pH 7.2–7.4, and sterilize by maintaining at 115 °C for 30 minutes.

Perchloric acid (~1170 g/l) TS [perchloric acid (70 per cent. w/w) R]. (SRIP, 1963, p. 137); $d \sim 1.67$.

Perchloric acid (~140 g/l) TS. Perchloric acid (~1170 g/l) TS, diluted with water to contain 141 g/l of $HClO_4$; $d \sim 1.09$.

Perchloric acid (0.1 mol/l) VS.
Procedure. To 900 ml of glacial acetic acid R1, at about 25 °C, add 8.2 ml of perchloric acid (~1170 g/l) TS, mix, add 32 ml of acetic anhydride R, and mix again. Cool to room temperature, add sufficient glacial acetic acid R1, to produce 1000 ml, and allow to stand for 24 hours.
Water. Determine the content by the Karl Fischer method. If necessary, add sufficient water or acetic anhydride R to adjust the content of water to between 0.1 and 2.0 mg/ml, and allow to stand for a further 24 hours.
Method of standardization. Ascertain the exact concentration by titrating 0.5 g, accurately weighed, of potassium hydrogen phthalate R, previously dried at 120 °C for 2 hours, using the Karl Fischer direct

titration method (Method A, see p. 135). Each ml of perchloric acid (0.1 mol/l) VS is equivalent to 20.42 mg of $C_8H_5KO_4$. Record the temperature at which the standardization is carried out.

Petroleum, light, R [light petroleum R]. (SRIP, 1963, p. 108).

o-Phenanthroline R. 1,10-Phenanthroline, $C_{12}H_8N_2,H_2O$ (SRIP, 1963, p. 138).

o-Phenanthroline (1 g/l) TS.
Procedure. Dissolve 0.11 g of o-phenanthroline R in sufficient water to produce 100 ml.

o-Phenanthroline TS.
Procedure. Dissolve 0.7 g of ferrous sulfate R in about 70 ml of water, add about 1.5 g of o-phenanthroline R and sufficient water to produce 100 ml.

Phenol R. C_6H_6O.
Description. Colourless, or at most faintly pink, cohering or separate acicular crystals, or crystalline masses; odour, characteristic. Corrosive, and blanches the skin and mucous membranes.
Solubility. Soluble in about 15 parts of water and in about 100 parts of liquid paraffin R; freely soluble in ethanol ($\sim$750 g/l) TS, ether R and chloroform R.
Completeness of solution. 1.0 g dissolves completely in 15 ml of water at 15 °C.
Congealing temperature. Not below 40.5 °C.
Residue on evaporation. Evaporate on a water-bath and dry to constant weight at 105 °C; leaves not more than 0.5 mg/g of residue.

Phenolphthalein R. $C_{20}H_{14}O_4$ (SRIP, 1963, p. 139).

Phenolphthalein/ethanol TS.
Procedure. Dissolve 1.0 g of phenolphthalein R in sufficient ethanol ($\sim$750 g/l) TS to produce 100 ml.

Phenolphthalein/pyridine TS.
Procedure. Dissolve 1.0 g of phenolphthalein R in sufficient pyridine R to produce 100 ml.

Phenol red R. Phenolsulfonphthalein, $C_{19}H_{14}O_5S$ (SRIP, 1963, p. 139).

Phenol red/ethanol TS.
Procedure. Dissolve 0.05 g of phenol red R in a mixture of 2.85 ml of sodium hydroxide (0.05 mol/l) VS and 5 ml of ethanol ($\sim$710 g/l) TS. Warm the solution slightly and after cooling dilute with sufficient ethanol ($\sim$150 g/l) TS to produce 250 ml.

Phosphate buffer, sterile, pH 4.5, TS.
Procedure. Dissolve 13.6 g of potassium dihydrogen phosphate R in sufficient water to produce 1000 ml. Sterilize the solution for

20 minutes in an autoclave at 120 °C and, if necessary, adjust the pH to 4.45–4.55 with phosphoric acid (~1440 g/l) TS or potassium hydroxide (~110 g/l) TS.

Phosphate buffer, sterile, pH 6.0, TS1.
Procedure. Dissolve 2.0 g of dipotassium hydrogen phosphate R and 8.0 g of potassium dihydrogen phosphate R in sufficient water to produce 1000 ml. Sterilize the solution for 20 minutes in an autoclave at 120 °C and, if necessary, adjust the pH to 5.95–6.05 with phosphoric acid (~1440 g/l) TS or potassium hydroxide (~110 g/l) TS.

Phosphate buffer, sterile, pH 6.0, TS2.
Procedure. Dissolve 1.16 g of anhydrous disodium hydrogen phosphate R and 7.96 g of potassium dihydrogen phosphate R in sufficient water to produce 1000 ml. Sterilize the solution for 20 minutes in an autoclave at 120 °C and, if necessary, adjust the pH to 5.95–6.05 with phosphoric acid (~1440 g/l) TS or potassium hydroxide (~110 g/l) TS.

Phosphate buffer, sterile, pH 6.0, TS3.
Procedure. Dissolve 20.0 g of dipotassium hydrogen phosphate R and 80.0 g of potassium dihydrogen phosphate R in sufficient water to produce 1000 ml. Sterilize the solution for 20 minutes in an autoclave at 120 °C and, if necessary, adjust the pH to 5.95–6.05 with phosphoric acid (~1440 g/l) TS or potassium hydroxide (~110 g/l) TS.

Phosphate standard buffer, pH 6.8, TS.
Procedure. Dissolve 3.40 g of potassium dihydrogen phosphate R and 3.53 g of anhydrous disodium hydrogen phosphate R in sufficient carbon-dioxide-free water R to produce 1000 ml.

Phosphate buffer, pH 7.0, TS.
Procedure. Dissolve 5.76 g of anhydrous disodium hydrogen phosphate R and 3.55 g of potassium dihydrogen phosphate R in sufficient water to produce 1000 ml.

Phosphate buffer, sterile, pH 7.0, TS.
Procedure. Dissolve 5.76 g of anhydrous disodium hydrogen phosphate R and 3.55 g of potassium dihydrogen phosphate R in sufficient water to produce 1000 ml. Sterilize the solution for 20 minutes in an autoclave at 120 °C and, if necessary, adjust the pH to 6.95–7.05 with phosphoric acid (~1440 g/l) TS or potassium hydroxide (~110 g/l) TS.

Phosphate buffer, sterile, pH 7.2, TS.
Procedure. Dissolve 6.80 g of potassium dihydrogen phosphate R and 1.4 g of sodium hydroxide R in sufficient water to produce 1000 ml. Sterilize the solution for 20 minutes in an autoclave at 120 °C and,

if necessary, adjust the pH to 7.1–7.3 with phosphoric acid (∼1440 g/l) TS or potassium hydroxide (∼110 g/l) TS.

Phosphate standard buffer, pH 7.4, TS.
Procedure. Dissolve 1.18 g of potassium dihydrogen phosphate R and 4.30 g of anhydrous disodium hydrogen phosphate R in sufficient carbon-dioxide-free water R to produce 1000 ml.

Phosphate buffer, sterile, pH 8.0, TS1.
Procedure. Dissolve 16.73 g of dipotassium hydrogen phosphate R and 0.52 g of potassium dihydrogen phosphate R in sufficient water to produce 1000 ml. Sterilize the solution for 20 minutes in an autoclave at 120 °C and, if necessary, adjust the pH to 7.9–8.1 with phosphoric acid (∼1440 g/l) TS or potassium hydroxide (∼110 g/l) TS.

Phosphate buffer, sterile, pH 8.0, TS2.
Procedure. Dissolve 8.95 g of anhydrous disodium hydrogen phosphate R and 0.50 g of potassium dihydrogen phosphate R in sufficient water to produce 1000 ml. Sterilize the solution for 20 minutes in an autoclave at 120 °C and, if necessary, adjust the pH to 7.9–8.1 with phosphoric acid (∼1440 g/l) TS or potassium hydroxide (∼110 g/l) TS.

Phosphoric acid (∼1440 g/l) TS [phosphoric acid R]. (SRIP, 1963, p. 141); $d \sim 1.7$.

Phosphorus pentoxide R. P_2O_5 (SRIP, 1963, p. 142).

Phthalic anhydride R. $C_8H_4O_3$.
Description. White lustrous needles.
Solubility. Slightly soluble in water, more soluble in hot water; soluble in ethanol (∼750 g/l) TS and ether R.
Melting temperature. About 130 °C.

Phthalic anhydride/pyridine TS.
Procedure. Add 42 g of phthalic anhydride R, accurately weighed, to 300 ml of freshly distilled pyridine R (refluxed with barium oxide R) containing less than 1 mg/ml of water in a glass-stoppered 1000 ml flask. Use a dark flask or otherwise prevent exposure to light. Shake vigorously until complete solution is effected, and allow to stand overnight for completion of the reaction.
Note: Phthalic anhydride/pyridine TS must be freshly prepared.

Polysorbate 80 R. The mono ester of oleic acid and tripolyethylene-glycol 300-sorbitan ether.
Description. Lemon to amber coloured, oily liquid.
Miscibility. Miscible with water, producing an odourless and nearly colourless solution. Miscible with ethanol (∼750 g/l) TS, ethyl acetate R, and vegetable oils; immiscible with mineral oils.

Potassium acetate R. $C_2H_3KO_2$ (SRIP, 1963, p. 144).

Potassium acetate TS.
Procedure. Dissolve 100 g of potassium acetate R in sufficient glacial acetic acid R to produce 1000 ml.

Potassium bicarbonate R. $KHCO_3$ (SRIP, 1963, p. 145).

Potassium bromide R. KBr (SRIP, 1963, p. 148).

Potassium bromide IR. Potassium bromide R that complies with the following test: The infrared absorption spectrum of a disc prepared as described in Method 3 under "Spectrophotometry in the infrared region" (see p. 41), from potassium bromide R, previously dried at 250 °C for 1 hour, has a substantially flat baseline over the range 4000–670 cm^{-1}; it exhibits no maxima with an absorbance greater than 0.1 above the baseline, with the exception of maxima due to water at 3440 and 1630 cm^{-1}.

Potassium bromide (100 g/l) TS. A solution of potassium bromide R containing about 100 g of KBr per litre.

Potassium chloride R. KCl (SRIP, 1963, p. 151).

Potassium chloride IR. Potassium chloride R that complies with the following test: The infrared absorption spectrum of a disc prepared as described in Method 3 under "Spectrophotometry in the infrared region" (see p. 41), from potassium chloride R, previously dried at 250 °C for 1 hour, has a substantially flat baseline over the range 4000–670 cm^{-1}; it exhibits no maxima with an absorbance greater than 0.1 above the baseline, with the exception of maxima due to water at 3440 and 1630 cm^{-1}.

Potassium chloride (350 g/l) TS. A saturated solution of potassium chloride R containing about 350 g/l of KCl.

Potassium dichromate R. $K_2Cr_2O_7$ (SRIP, 1963, p. 154).

Potassium dichromate R1. Potassium dichromate R containing not less than 99.9 % of $K_2Cr_2O_7$.

Potassium dichromate TS.
Procedure. Dissolve about 60 mg, accurately weighed and previously dried at 130 °C, of potassium dichromate R1 in sufficient sulfuric acid (0.005 mol/l) VS to produce 1000.0 ml.

Potassium dichromate (0.0167 mol/l) VS. Potassium dichromate R, dissolved in water to contain 4.904 g of $K_2Cr_2O_7$ in 1000 ml.

Potassium dihydrogen phosphate R. KH_2PO_4 (SPRI, 1963, p. 155).

Potassium ferricyanide R. $K_3Fe(CN)_6$ (SRIP, 1963, p. 156).

Potassium ferricyanide (10 g/l) TS.

Procedure. Wash about 1 g of crystalline potassium ferricyanide R with a little water and dissolve the washed crystals in sufficient water to produce 100 ml.

Note: Potassium ferricyanide (10 g/l) TS must be freshly prepared.

Potassium hydrogen phthalate R. $C_8H_5KO_4$ (SRIP, 1963, p. 157).

Potassium hydrogen phthalate standard TS.

Procedure. Dissolve 10.21 g of potassium hydrogen phthalate R, previously dried at 120 °C, in sufficient carbon-dioxide-free water R to produce 1000 ml. The pH of this solution is defined as having the value of 4.000 at 15 °C.

Potassium hydrogen tartrate R. $C_4H_5KO_6$ (SRIP, 1963, p. 158).

Potassium hydrogen tartrate standard TS.

Procedure. Add 2 g of potassium hydrogen tartrate R to 100 ml of carbon-dioxide-free water R contained in a glass-stoppered flask and shake the flask vigorously. Let the temperature of the solution reach room temperature, allow the solid to settle, and remove it by filtration or decantation.

Note: Potassium hydrogen tartrate standard TS must be freshly prepared.

Potassium hydroxide R. KOH (SRIP, 1963, p. 159).

Potassium hydroxide (∼110 g/l) TS. A solution of potassium hydroxide R containing about 112 g/l of KOH (approximately 2 mol/l).

Potassium hydroxide/ethanol TS1.

Procedure. Dissolve 40 g of potassium hydroxide R in 20 ml of water and add sufficient ethanol (∼750 g/l) TS to produce 1000 ml. Allow to stand overnight, and pour off the clear liquid.

Potassium hydroxide (1 mol/l) VS. Potassium hydroxide R, dissolved in water to contain 56.10 g of KOH in 1000 ml.

Method of standardization. Ascertain the exact concentration of the 1 mol/l solution in the following manner: Dry about 5 g of potassium hydrogen phthalate R at 105 °C for 3 hours and weigh accurately. If the potassium hydrogen phthalate is in the form of large crystals, they should be crushed before drying. Dissolve in 75 ml of carbon-dioxide-free water R and titrate with the potassium hydroxide solution, using phenolphthalein/ethanol TS as indicator. Each 0.2042 g of potassium hydrogen phthalate is equivalent to 1 ml of potassium hydroxide (1 mol/l) VS. Standard solutions of potassium hydroxide should be restandardized frequently.

Storage. Solutions of alkali hydroxides absorb carbon dioxide when exposed to air. They should therefore be stored in bottles with suitable non-glass, well-fitting stoppers, provided with a tube filled with soda lime R.

Potassium hydroxide (0.5 mol/l) VS.   Potassium hydroxide R, dissolved in water to contain 28.05 g of KOH in 1000 ml.
Method of standardization.   Ascertain the exact concentration of the solution following the method described under potassium hydroxide (1 mol/l) VS.

Potassium hydroxide (0.1 mol/l) VS.   Potassium hydroxide R, dissolved in water to contain 5.610 g of KOH in 1000 ml.
Method of standardization.   Ascertain the exact concentration of the solution following the method described under potassium hydroxide (1 mol/l) VS.

Potassium hydroxide/ethanol (0.5 mol/l) VS.   Potassium hydroxide R, dissolved in ethanol ($\sim$710 g/l) TS to contain 28.05 g of KOH in 1000 ml.
Method of standardization.   Ascertain the exact concentration of the 0.5 mol/l solution in the following manner: Dilute 25.0 ml of hydrochloric acid (0.5 mol/l) VS with 50 ml of water and titrate with the potassium hydroxide/ethanol solution, using phenolphthalein/ethanol TS as indicator.

Potassium hydroxide/ethanol (0.02 mol/l) VS.   Potassium hydroxide R, dissolved in ethanol ($\sim$710 g/l) TS to contain 1.122 g of KOH in 1000 ml.
Method of standardization.   Ascertain the exact concentration of the solution following the method described under potassium hydroxide/ethanol (0.5 mol/l) VS.

Potassium iodide R.   KI (SRIP, 1963, p. 161).

Potassium iodide AsR.   Potassium iodide R that complies with the following test: Dissolve 10 g of potassium iodide R in 25 ml of hydrochloric acid ($\sim$250 g/l) AsTS and 35 ml of water, add 2 drops of stannous chloride AsTS and apply the general test for arsenic; no visible stain is produced.

Potassium iodide (80 g/l) TS.   A solution of potassium iodide R containing about 83 g/l of KI (approximately 0.5 mol/l).

Potassium nitrate R. KNO_3 (SRIP, 1963, p. 162).

Potassium nitrite R. KNO_2.
Description.   White or slightly yellow, deliquescent granules or rods.
Solubility.   Soluble in 0.35 part of water; slightly soluble in ethanol ($\sim$750 g/l) TS.

Potassium nitrite (100 g/l) TS.   A solution of potassium nitrite R containing about 100 g/l of KNO_2.

Potassium permanganate R. $KMnO_4$ (SRIP, 1963, p. 165).

Potassium permanganate (10 g/l) TS. A solution of potassium permanganate R containing about 10 g/l of $KMnO_4$.

Potassium permanganate (0.02 mol/l) VS. Potassium permanganate R, dissolved in water to contain 3.161 g of $KMnO_4$ in 1000 ml.
Method of standardization. Ascertain the exact concentration of the 0.02 mol/l solution in the following manner: Dissolve about 0.2 g, accurately weighed, of sodium oxalate R, previously dried to constant weight at 110 °C, in 250 ml of water. Add 7 ml of sulfuric acid (~1760 g/l) TS, heat to about 70 °C and then slowly add the permanganate solution from a burette, with constant stirring, until a pale pink colour, which persists for 15 seconds, is produced. The temperature at the conclusion of the titration should be not less than 60 °C. Every 6.7 mg of sodium oxalate are equivalent to 1 ml of potassium permanganate (0.02 mol/l) VS. Potassium permanganate solutions should be restandardized frequently.
Storage. Store the solution in tightly closed containers, protected from light.

Potassium sulfate R. K_2SO_4 (SRIP, 1963, p. 165).

Potassium sulfate (174 mg/l) TS.
Procedure. Dissolve 174 mg, accurately weighed, of potassium sulfate R in sufficient water to produce 1000 ml.

Potassium tetraoxalate R. $C_4H_3KO_8,2H_2O$ (SRIP, 1963, p. 166).

Potassium tetraoxalate standard TS.
Procedure. Dissolve 25.42 g of potassium tetraoxalate R in sufficient carbon-dioxide-free water R to produce 1000 ml.

Pyridine R. C_5H_5N (SRIP, 1963, p. 169).

Pyridine, anhydrous, R. Pyridine R that has been dried by allowing it to stand over sodium hydroxide R.

Red stock standard TS.
Procedure. To 40.4 ml of cobalt colour TS, add 6.1 ml of copper colour TS, 6.3 ml of dichromate colour TS, 12.0 ml of iron colour TS, dilute to 100.0 ml with sulfuric acid (~10 g/l) TS, and mix.

Resazurin sodium R. $C_{12}H_6NNaO_4$ (SRIP, 1963, p. 170).

Resazurin sodium (1 g/l) TS. A solution of resazurin sodium R containing about 1 g/l of $C_{12}H_6NNaO_4$.
Note: Resazurin sodium (1 g/l) TS must be freshly prepared.

Resorcinol R. 1,3-Dihydroxybenzene, $C_6H_6O_2$ (SRIP, 1963, p. 171).

Resorcinol (20 g/l) TS. A solution of resorcinol R containing 20 g/l of $C_6H_6O_2$.

Saline TS. A sterile solution of sodium chloride R containing about 9 g/l of NaCl. Sterilization by heating in a steam autoclave at 120 °C for 30 minutes is suitable.

Selenium R. Se (SRIP, 1963, p. 172).
Caution. Selenium vapours are toxic.

Silica gel, desiccant, R.
Description. An amorphous, partly hydrated SiO_2, occurring in glassy granules of varying sizes. It is frequently coated with a substance that changes colour when the capacity to absorb water is exhausted. Such coloured products may be regenerated (i.e., may regain their capacity to absorb water) by heating at 110 °C until the gel assumes the original colour.
Loss on ignition. Ignite 2 g, accurately weighed, at 950 ± 50 °C to constant weight; the loss is not more than 60 mg/g.
Water absorption. Place about 10 g in a tared weighing-bottle, and weigh. Then place the bottle, with the cover removed, for 24 hours in a closed container in which the atmosphere is maintained at 80 % relative humidity by being in equilibrium with sulfuric acid having a relative density of 1.19. Weigh again; the increase in weight is not less than 310 mg/g.

Silver nitrate R. $AgNO_3$ (SRIP, 1963, p. 173).

Silver nitrate (40 g/l) TS. A solution of silver nitrate R containing about 42.5 g/l of $AgNO_3$ (approximately 0.25 mol/l).

Silver nitrate (0.1 mol/l) VS. Silver nitrate R, dissolved in water to contain 16.99 g of $AgNO_3$ in 1000 ml.
Method of standardization. Ascertain the exact concentration of the 0.1 mol/l solution in the following manner: Dilute 40.0 ml of the silver nitrate solution with 100 ml of water. Heat the solution and add slowly, with continuous stirring, hydrochloric acid (∼70 g/l) TS until precipitation of the silver is complete. Boil the mixture cautiously for about 5 minutes, then allow it to stand in the dark until the precipitate has settled and the supernatant liquid has become clear. Transfer the precipitate completely to a tared filtering crucible and wash it with small portions of water that has been slightly acidified with nitric acid (∼1000 g/l) TS. Dry the precipitate to constant weight at 110 °C. From the weight of silver chloride calculate the concentration of the silver nitrate solution in mol/l. Protect the silver chloride from light as much as possible during the determination.

Soda lime R. (SRIP, 1963, p. 174).

Sodium acetate R. $C_2H_3NaO_2,3H_2O$ (SRIP, 1963, p. 176).

Sodium acetate (150 g/l) TS. A solution of sodium acetate R containing about 150 g/l of $C_2H_3NaO_2$.

Sodium alizarinsulfonate R. Alizarin Red S, sodium salt of 3,4-dihydroxy-9,10-anthraquinone-2-sulfonic acid; $C_{14}H_7NaO_7S,H_2O$.
Description. A yellow-brown or orange-yellow powder.
Solubility. Freely soluble in water, producing a yellow solution; sparingly soluble in ethanol ($\sim$750 g/l) TS.

Sodium alizarinsulfonate (1 g/l) TS.
Procedure. Dissolve 0.11 g of sodium alizarinsulfonate R in sufficient water to produce 100 ml.

Sodium bicarbonate R. $NaHCO_3$ (SRIP, 1963, p. 177).

Sodium carbonate R. $Na_2CO_3,10H_2O$ (SRIP, 1963, p. 179).

Sodium carbonate, anhydrous, R. Na_2CO_3 (SRIP, 1963, p. 179).

Sodium carbonate (50 g/l) TS. A solution of sodium carbonate R containing about 50 g/l of Na_2CO_3 (approximately 0.5 mol/l).

Sodium carbonate standard TS.
Procedure. Dissolve 2.64 g of sodium carbonate R and 2.093 g of sodium bicarbonate R in sufficient carbon-dioxide-free water R to produce 1000 ml.

Sodium chloride R. NaCl (SRIP, 1963, p. 181).

Sodium citrate R. $C_6H_5Na_3O_7,2H_2O$.
Contains not less than 99.0 % of $C_6H_5Na_3O_7$, calculated with reference to the anhydrous substance.
Description. White, granular crystals or a crystalline powder; odourless. Slightly deliquescent in moist air.
Solubility. Soluble in less than 2 parts of water, practically insoluble in ethanol ($\sim$750 g/l) TS.
Appearance of solution. A 100 g/l solution is clear and colourless.
Water. Determined by the Karl Fischer method, keeping the substance in contact with the dehydrated methanol R for 15 minutes; not less than 110 mg/g and not more than 130 mg/g.
Assay. Dissolve about 0.15 g, accurately weighed, in 20 ml of glacial acetic acid R, and titrate with perchloric acid (0.1 mol/l) VS as described in "Non-aqueous Titration", Method A (see p. 131). Each ml of perchloric acid (0.1 mol/l) VS is equivalent to 8.603 mg of $C_6H_5Na_3O_7$.

Sodium cobaltinitrite R. $Na_3Co(NO_2)_6$ (SRIP, 1963, p. 182).

Sodium cobaltinitrite (100 g/l) TS. A solution of sodium cobaltinitrite R containing about 100 g/l of $Na_3Co(NO_2)_6$.

Sodium fluoride R. NaF (SRIP, 1963, p. 183).

Sodium hydroxide R. NaOH (SRIP, 1963, p. 185).

Sodium hydroxide ($\sim$400 g/l) TS. A solution of sodium hydroxide R containing about 400 g/l of NaOH.

Sodium hydroxide (~300 g/l) TS. A solution of sodium hydroxide R containing about 300 g/l of NaOH.

Sodium hydroxide (~200 g/l) TS. A solution of sodium hydroxide R containing about 200 g/l of NaOH.

Sodium hydroxide (~80 g/l) TS. A solution of sodium hydroxide R containing about 80 g/l of NaOH (approximately 2 mol/l).

Sodium hydroxide (1 mol/l) VS. Sodium hydroxide R, dissolved in water to contain 40.01 g of NaOH in 1000 ml.

Method of standardization. Ascertain the exact concentration of the 1 mol/l solution in the following manner: Dry about 5 g of potassium hydrogen phthalate R at 105 °C for 3 hours and weigh accurately. If the potassium hydrogen phthalate is in the form of large crystals, they should be crushed before drying. Dissolve in 75 ml of carbon-dioxide-free water R and titrate with the sodium hydroxide solution, using phenolphthalein/ethanol TS as indicator. Each 0.2042 g of potassium hydrogen phthalate is equivalent to 1 ml of sodium hydroxide (1 mol/l) VS. Standard solutions of sodium hydroxide should be restandardized frequently.

Storage. Solutions of alkali hydroxides absorb carbon dioxide when exposed to air. They should therefore be stored in bottles with suitable non-glass, well-fitting stoppers, provided with a tube filled with soda lime R.

Sodium hydroxide (0.2 mol/l) VS. Sodium hydroxide R, dissolved in water to contain 8.001 g of NaOH in 1000 ml.

Method of standardization. Ascertain the exact concentration of the solution following the method described under sodium hydroxide (1 mol/l) VS.

Sodium hydroxide (0.1 mol/l) VS. Sodium hydroxide R, dissolved in water to contain 4.001 g of NaOH in 1000 ml.

Method of standardization. Ascertain the exact concentration of the solution following the method described under sodium hydroxide (1 mol/l) VS.

Sodium hydroxide (0.05 mol/l) VS. Sodium hydroxide R, dissolved in water to contain 2.000 g of NaOH in 1000 ml.

Method of standardization. Ascertain the exact concentration of the solution following the method described under sodium hydroxide (1 mol/l) VS.

Sodium hydroxide (0.01 mol/l) VS. Sodium hydroxide R, dissolved in water to contain 0.4001 g of NaOH in 1000 ml.

Method of standardization. Ascertain the exact concentration of the solution following the method described under sodium hydroxide (1 mol/l) VS.

Sodium hydroxide (1 mol/l), carbonate-free, VS. Sodium hydroxide R, dissolved in water to contain 40.01 g of NaOH in 1000 ml.

Procedure. Dissolve sodium hydroxide R in water to produce a 400–600 g/l solution and allow to stand. Taking precautions to avoid absorption of carbon dioxide, siphon off the clear supernatant liquid and dilute as required with carbon-dioxide-free water R.

Test for carbonates. Titrate 45 ml of hydrochloric acid (1 mol/l) VS with the carbonate-free sodium hydroxide solution, using phenolphthalein/ethanol TS as indicator. At the endpoint add just sufficient acid to discharge the pink colour and boil to reduce the volume to 20 ml. Add, whilst boiling, sufficient acid again to discharge the pink colour and prevent its reappearance on continued boiling; not more than 0.1 ml of the acid is required.

Method of standardization. Ascertain the exact concentration of the 1 mol/l solution in the following manner: Dry about 5 g of potassium hydrogen phthalate R at 105 °C for 3 hours and weigh accurately. If the potassium hydrogen phthalate is in the form of large crystals, they should be crushed before drying. Dissolve in 75 ml of carbon-dioxide-free water R and titrate with the carbonate-free sodium hydroxide solution, using phenolphthalein/ethanol TS as indicator. Each 0.2042 g of potassium hydrogen phthalate is equivalent to 1 ml of carbonate-free sodium hydroxide (1 mol/l) VS. Standard solutions of sodium hydroxide should be restandardized frequently.

Storage. Solutions of alkali hydroxides absorb carbon dioxide when exposed to air They should therefore be stored in bottles with suitable non-glass, well-fitting stoppers, provided with a tube filled with soda lime R.

Sodium hydroxide (0.5 mol/l), carbonate-free, VS. Sodium hydroxide R, dissolved in water to contain 20.00 g of NaOH in 1000 ml.

Procedure, test for carbonates and method of standardization. Prepare the solution, carry out the test, and ascertain the exact concentration following the method described under carbonate-free sodium hydroxide (1 mol/l) VS.

Sodium hydroxide (0.2 mol/l), carbonate-free, VS. Sodium hydroxide R, dissolved in water to contain 8.001 g of NaOH in 1000 ml.

Procedure, test for carbonates and method of standardization. Prepare the solution, carry out the test, and ascertain the exact concentration following the method described under carbonate-free sodium hydroxide (1 mol/l) VS.

Sodium hydroxide (0.1 mol/l), carbonate-free, VS. Sodium hydroxide R, dissolved in water to contain 4.001 g of NaOH in 1000 ml.

Procedure, test for carbonates and method of standardization. Prepare the solution, carry out the test, and ascertain the exact concentration following the method described under carbonate-free sodium hydroxide (1 mol/l) VS.

Sodium hydroxide (0.02 mol/l), carbonate-free, VS. Sodium hydroxide R, dissolved in water to contain 0.8001 g of NaOH in 1000 ml.
Procedure, test for carbonates and method of standardization. Prepare the solution, carry out the test, and ascertain the exact concentration following the method described under carbonate-free sodium hydroxide (1 mol/l) VS.

Sodium hydroxide (0.01 mol/l), carbonate-free, VS. Sodium hydroxide R, dissolved in water to contain 0.4001 g of NaOH in 1000 ml.
Procedure, test for carbonates and method of standardization. Prepare the solution, carry out the test, and ascertain the exact concentration following the method described under carbonate-free sodium hydroxide (1 mol/l) VS.

Sodium mercaptoacetate R. (Sodium thioglycolate R.) $C_2H_3NaO_2S$.
Description. Hygroscopic crystals.
Solubility. Freely soluble in water; slightly soluble in ethanol ($\sim$750 g/l) TS.

Sodium nitrite R. $NaNO_2$ (SRIP, 1963, p. 189).

Sodium nitrite (10 g/l) TS. A solution of sodium nitrite R containing about 10 g/l of $NaNO_2$.

Sodium nitrite (0.1 mol/l) VS. Sodium nitrite R, dissolved in water to contain 6.900 g of $NaNO_2$ in 1000 ml.
Method of standardization. Ascertain the exact concentration of the 0.1 mol/l solution in the following manner: Place 50.0 ml of potassium permanganate (0.02 mol/l) VS in a glass-stoppered flask, dilute with 300 ml of water, add 25 ml of sulfuric acid ($\sim$100 g/l) TS and 20.0 ml of the sodium nitrite solution. Allow the solution to stand for 10 minutes. Then add 2 g of potassium iodide R and titrate with sodium thiosulfate (0.1 mol/l) VS, using starch TS as indicator. Perform a blank determination and make any necessary corrections.

Sodium oxalate R. $C_2Na_2O_4$ (SRIP, 1963, p. 190).

Sodium sulfate, anhydrous, R. Na_2SO_4 (SRIP, 1963, p. 195).

Sodium sulfide R. $Na_2S,9H_2O$ (SRIP, 1963, p. 195).

Sodium sulfide TS.
Procedure. Dissolve 12 g of sodium sulfide R in 25 ml of water and add sufficient glycerol R to produce 100 ml.

Sodium tetraborate R. Borax, $Na_2B_4O_7$, 10 H_2O.
Description. Transparent, colourless crystals, or a white, crystalline powder; odourless.

Solubility. Soluble in 20 parts of water, and in 0.6 part of boiling water; very slightly soluble in ethanol ($\sim$750 g/l) TS.

pH Value of a 0.01 mol/l solution. Dissolve 0.3814 g in water and dilute to 100 ml, using water having a pH of 6.5–7.4. The pH should be from 9.15–9.20 at 25 °C.

Chlorides. Dissolve 1.0 g in 20 ml of water, filter if necessary through a chloride-free filter, add 1 ml of nitric acid ($\sim$1000 g/l) TS, and proceed as described in " Limit test for chlorides " (see p. 115). Sodium tetraborate R contains not more than 250 μg/g.

Sulfates. Dissolve 0.5 g in 20 ml of water, add 2 ml of hydrochloric acid ($\sim$70 g/l) TS, and filter. Proceed as described in "Limit test for sulfates" (see p. 116). Sodium tetraborate R contains not more than 1.0 mg/g.

Sodium tetraborate standard TS.

Procedure. Dissolve 3.81 g of sodium tetraborate R in sufficient carbon-dioxide-free water R to produce 1000 ml.

Storage. Store the solution protected from atmospheric carbon dioxide and keep it stoppered at all times except when actually in use.

Sodium tetraphenylborate R. $C_{24}H_{20}BNa$.

Description. A fluffy, white or almost white powder.

Solubility. Freely soluble in water and acetone R; insoluble in light petroleum R.

pH Value. pH of a 20 g/l solution, not less than 7.5.

Sodium tetraphenylborate (30 g/l) TS. A solution of sodium tetraphenyl-borate R containing about 30 g/l of $C_{24}H_{20}BNa$.

Note: If necessary, stir for 5 minutes with 1 g of aluminium hydroxide R or charcoal R, and filter to clarify.

Sodium thioglycolate R. *See* **Sodium mercaptoacetate R.**

Sodium thiosulfate R. $Na_2S_2O_3$, 5 H_2O (SRIP, 1963, p. 197).

Sodium thiosulfate (0.1 mol/l) VS. Sodium thiosulfate R, dissolved in water to contain 15.82 g of $Na_2S_2O_3$ in 1000 ml.

Method of standardization. Ascertain the exact concentration of the 0.1 mol/l solution in the following manner: Transfer 30.0 ml of potassium dichromate (0.0167 mol/l) VS to a glass-stoppered flask and dilute with 50 ml of water. Add 2 g of potassium iodide R and 5 ml of hydrochloric acid ($\sim$250 g/l) TS, stopper and allow to stand for 10 minutes. Dilute with 100 ml of water and titrate the liberated iodine with the sodium thiosulfate solution, using starch TS as indicator. Sodium thiosulfate solutions should be restandardized frequently.

Sodium thiosulfate (0.05 mol/l) VS. Sodium thiosulfate R, dissolved in water to contain 7.910 g of $Na_2S_2O_3$ in 1000 ml.

Method of standardization. Ascertain the exact concentration of the solution by following the method described under sodium thiosulfate (0.1 mol/l) VS.

Sodium thiosulfate (0.01 mol/l) VS. Sodium thiosulfate R, dissolved in water to contain 1.582 g of $Na_2S_2O_3$ in 1000 ml.

Method of standardization. Ascertain the exact concentration of the solution by following the method described under sodium thiosulfate (0.1 mol/l) VS.

Stannous chloride R. $SnCl_2,2H_2O$ (SRIP, 1963, p. 198).

Stannous chloride TS.
Procedure. Dissolve 330 g of stannous chloride R in 100 ml of hydrochloric acid ($\sim$250 g/l) TS and sufficient water to produce 1000 ml.

Stannous chloride AsTS.
Procedure. Prepare from stannous chloride TS by adding an equal volume of hydrochloric acid ($\sim$250 g/l) TS, boil down to the original volume, and filter through a fine-grained filter-paper.
Test for arsenic. To 10 ml add 6 ml of water and 10 ml of hydrochloric acid ($\sim$250 g/l) AsTS, and distil 16 ml. To the distillate add 50 ml of water and 2 drops of stannous chloride AsTS; then apply the general test for arsenic. The colour of the stain produced is not more intense than that produced from a 1-ml standard stain, showing that the amount of arsenic does not exceed 1 μg/ml.

Starch R [potato starch R or corn starch R]. (SRIP, 1963, p. 199).

Starch, soluble, R. (SRIP, 1963, p. 199).

Starch TS.
Procedure. Mix 0.5 g of starch R or of soluble starch R with 5 ml of water, and add this solution, with constant stirring, to sufficient water to produce about 100 ml; boil for a few minutes, cool, and filter.
Note: Starch TS must be freshly prepared.

Starch/iodide paper R [starch-iodide paper R]. (SRIP, 1963, p. 200).

Sulfosalicylic acid R. $C_7H_6O_6S,2H_2O$.
Description. White or slightly pink coloured, needle-like crystals.
Solubility. Soluble in water and ethanol ($\sim$750 g/l) TS.
Insoluble matter. Dissolve 5.0 g in 50 ml of water, heat to boiling and digest in a covered beaker on a water-bath for 1 hour. Filter through a tared filtering crucible, wash thoroughly, and dry at 105 °C. The weight of the residue does not exceed 1.0 mg.
Sulfated ash. Gently ignite 1.0 g in a tared crucible or dish, other

than platinum, until charred. Cool, moisten the residue with 1 ml of sulfuric acid ($\sim$1760 g/l) TS, and ignite again; not more than 1.0 mg/g.

Sulfosalicylic acid (175 g/l) TS. A solution of sulfosalicylic acid R containing about 175 g/l of $C_7H_6O_6S$.

Sulfur dioxide R. SO_2 (SRIP, 1963, p. 202).

Sulfuric acid ($\sim$1760 g/l) TS [sulfuric acid R]. (SRIP, 1963, p. 202); $d \sim 1.84$.

Sulfuric acid ($\sim$1760 g/l), nitrogen-free, TS. Sulfuric acid ($\sim$1760 g/l) TS containing not less than 1760 g/l of H_2SO_4 and complying with the test for nitrates.

Nitrates. Mix 45 ml with 5 ml of water, cool, and add 8 mg of diphenyl-benzidine R; the solution is colourless or not more than very pale blue.

Sulfuric acid ($\sim$190 g/l) TS.

Procedure. Mix 1 volume of sulfuric acid ($\sim$1760 g/l) TS with 9 volumes of water, and cool. The resulting solution contains about 190 g/l of H_2SO_4; $d \sim 1.12$.

Sulfuric acid ($\sim$100 g/l) TS.

Procedure. Add 57 ml of sulfuric acid ($\sim$1760 g/l) TS to sufficient water to produce 1000 ml (approximately 1 mol/l); $d \sim 1.065$.

Sulfuric acid ($\sim$10 g/l) TS.

Procedure. Mix 100 ml of sulfuric acid ($\sim$100 g/l) TS with sufficient water to produce 1000 ml.

Sulfuric acid (0.5 mol/l) VS. Sulfuric acid ($\sim$1760 g/l) TS, diluted with water to contain 49.04 g of H_2SO_4 in 1000 ml.

Method of standardization. Ascertain the exact concentration of the 0.5 mol/l solution in the following manner: Dissolve about 1.5 g, accurately weighed, of anhydrous sodium carbonate R, previously dried at 270 °C for 1 hour, in 50 ml of water and titrate with the sulfuric acid solution, using methyl orange/ethanol TS as indicator. Each 52.99 mg of anhydrous sodium carbonate is equivalent to 1 ml of sulfuric acid (0.5 mol/l) VS.

Sulfuric acid (0.05 mol/l) VS. Sulfuric acid ($\sim$1760 g/l) TS, diluted with water to contain 4.904 g of H_2SO_4 in 1000 ml.

Method of standardization. Ascertain the exact concentration of the solution following the method described under sulfuric acid (0.5 mol/l) VS.

Sulfuric acid (0.01 mol/l) VS. Sulfuric acid ($\sim$1760 g/l) TS, diluted with water to contain 0.9808 g of H_2SO_4 in 1000 ml.

Method of standardization. Ascertain the exact concentration of the solution following the method described under sulfuric acid (0.5 mol/l) VS.

Sulfuric acid (0.005 mol/l) VS. Sulfuric acid ($\sim$1760 g/l) TS, diluted with water to contain 0.4904 g of H_2SO_4 in 1000 ml.
Method of standardization. Ascertain the exact concentration of the solution following the method described under sulfuric acid (0.5 mol/l) VS.

p-**Terphenyl R.** 1,4-Diphenylbenzene, $C_{18}H_{14}$. Suitable for scintillation counting.

Thioglycolic acid R. *See* **Mercaptoacetic acid R.**

Thorin R. 2,7-Disodium 4-[(*o*-arsonophenyl)azo]-3-hydroxy-2,7-naph-thalenedisulfonate, $C_{16}H_{11}AsN_2Na_2O_{10}S_2$.

Thorin (2 g/l) TS.
Procedure. Dissolve 0.2 g of thorin R in sufficient water to produce 100 ml.
Storage. Store the solution protected from light.
Shelf-life. Use within 1 week of preparation.

Thorium nitrate R. $Th(NO_3)_4,4H_2O$.
Description. White, slightly deliquescent crystals.
Solubility. Very soluble in water and ethanol ($\sim$750 g/l) TS.

Thorium nitrate (0.005 mol/l) VS. Thorium nitrate R, dissolved in water to contain 2.401 g of $Th(NO_3)_4$ in 1000 ml.
Method of standardization. Ascertain the exact concentration of the 0.005 mol/l solution in the following manner: Transfer 0.050 g, accurately weighed, of sodium fluoride R, previously dried, to a flask and dissolve in sufficient water to produce 250 ml. To 20.0 ml of this solution add 0.6 ml of sodium alizarinsulfonate (1 g/l) TS and then, by drops, sodium hydroxide (0.1 mol/l) VS until the colour changes from pink to yellow. Add 5 ml of acetate buffer, pH 3.0, TS and titrate with the thorium nitrate solution until the yellow colour changes to pinkish yellow. Each 0.8398 mg of sodium fluoride is equivalent to 1 ml of thorium nitrate (0.005 mol/l) VS.

Thymolphthalein R. $C_{28}H_{30}O_4$ (SRIP, 1963, p. 207).

Thymolphthalein/ethanol TS.
Procedure. Dissolve 0.1 g of thymolphthalein R in 100 ml of ethanol ($\sim$750 g/l) TS, and filter if necessary.

Toluene R. C_7H_8 (SRIP, 1963, p. 209).

Uranyl acetate R. $C_4H_6O_6U$, 2 H_2O (SRIP, 1963, p. 213).
Uranyl/zinc acetate TS.
Procedure. Dissolve 10 g of uranyl acetate R by heating with 50 ml of water and 5 ml of acetic acid ($\sim$300 g/l) TS; dissolve 30 g of zinc

acetate R by heating with 30 ml of water and 3 ml of acetic acid (∼300 g/l) TS. Mix the two solutions, allow to cool to room temperature, and remove by filtration any solid material that separates.

Water, carbon-dioxide-free, R. Water that has been boiled vigorously for a few minutes and protected from the atmosphere during cooling and storage.

Xylenol orange R [3H-2,1-Benzoxathiol-3-ylidene bis[(6-hydroxy-5-methyl-m-phenylene)methylenenitrilo]]tetraacetic acid, S,S-dioxide, $C_{31}H_{32}N_2O_{13}S$.
Description. An orange powder.
Solubility. Soluble in water and ethanol (∼750 g/l) TS.

Xylenol orange indicator mixture R.
Procedure. Mix 0.1 g of xylenol orange R with 10 g of potassium nitrate R.

Yeast extract, water-soluble, R. (SRIP, 1963, p. 215).

Yellow stock standard TS.
Procedure. To 9.5 ml of cobalt colour TS, add 1.9 ml of copper colour TS, 10.7 ml of dichromate colour TS, 4.0 ml of iron colour TS, dilute to 100.0 ml with sulfuric acid (∼10 g/l) TS, and mix.

Zinc R. Zn (SRIP, 1963, p. 216); granulated, powder, or dust.

Zinc AsR, granulated. Granulated zinc R that complies with the following tests:
Limit of arsenic. Add 10 ml of stannated hydrochloric acid (∼250 g/l) AsTS to 50 ml of water, and apply the general test for arsenic; use 10 g of granulated zinc R and allow the reaction to continue for 1 hour; no visible stain is produced.
Test for sensitivity. Repeat the test for arsenic with the addition of 0.1 ml of dilute arsenic AsTS; a faint, but distinct yellow coloured stain is produced.

Zinc acetate R. $C_4H_6O_4Zn,2H_2O$ (SRIP, 1963, p. 216).

INDEX

INDEX